Department of Veterans Affairs
Health Services Research & Development Service

Evidence-based Synthesis Program

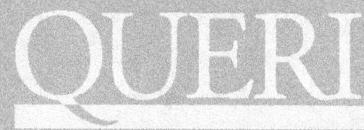

Effects of Health Plan-Sponsored Fitness Center Benefits on Physical Activity, Health Outcomes, and Health Care Costs and Utilization: A Systematic Review

October 2012

Prepared for:
Department of Veterans Affairs
Veterans Health Administration
Quality Enhancement Research Initiative
Health Services Research & Development Service
Washington, DC 20420

Prepared by:
Evidence-based Synthesis Program (ESP) Center
Durham VA Medical Center
Durham, NC
John W Williams Jr., M.D., M.H.Sc., Director

Investigators:
Co-Principal Investigators:
Heather A. King, Ph.D.
Jennifer M. Gierisch, Ph.D., M.P.H.

Co-Investigators:
John W. Williams Jr., M.D., M.H.Sc.
Matthew L. Maciejewski, Ph.D.

Research Associate:
Avishek Nagi, M.S.

Medical Editor:
Liz Wing, M.A.

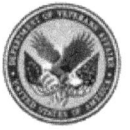 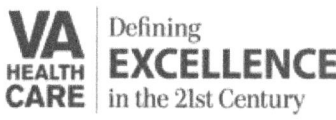

PREFACE

Quality Enhancement Research Initiative's (QUERI's) Evidence-based Synthesis Program (ESP) was established to provide timely and accurate syntheses of targeted healthcare topics of particular importance to Veterans Affairs (VA) managers and policymakers, as they work to improve the health and healthcare of Veterans. The ESP disseminates these reports throughout VA.

QUERI provides funding for four ESP Centers and each Center has an active VA affiliation. The ESP Centers generate evidence syntheses on important clinical practice topics, and these reports help:
- develop clinical policies informed by evidence,
- guide the implementation of effective services to improve patient outcomes and to support VA clinical practice guidelines and performance measures, and
- set the direction for future research to address gaps in clinical knowledge.

In 2009, the ESP Coordinating Center was created to expand the capacity of QUERI Central Office and the four ESP sites by developing and maintaining program processes. In addition, the Center established a Steering Committee comprised of QUERI field-based investigators, VA Patient Care Services, Office of Quality and Performance, and Veterans Integrated Service Networks (VISN) Clinical Management Officers. The Steering Committee provides program oversight, guides strategic planning, coordinates dissemination activities, and develops collaborations with VA leadership to identify new ESP topics of importance to Veterans and the VA healthcare system.

Comments on this evidence report are welcome and can be sent to Nicole Floyd, ESP Coordinating Center Program Manager, at nicole.floyd@va.gov.

Recommended citation: King HA, Gierisch JM, Williams JW Jr, Maciejewski ML. Effects of Health Plan-Sponsored Fitness Center Benefits on Physical Activity, Health Outcomes, and Health Care Costs and Utilization: A Systematic Review. VA-ESP Project #09-010; 2012.

This report is based on research conducted by the Evidence-based Synthesis Program (ESP) Center located at the Durham VA Medical Center, Durham, NC, funded by the Department of Veterans Affairs, Veterans Health Administration, Office of Research and Development, Health Services Research and Development. The findings and conclusions in this document are those of the author(s) who are responsible for its contents; the findings and conclusions do not necessarily represent the views of the Department of Veterans Affairs or the United States government. Therefore, no statement in this article should be construed as an official position of the Department of Veterans Affairs. No investigators have any affiliations or financial involvement (e.g., employment, consultancies, honoraria, stock ownership or options, expert testimony, grants or patents received or pending, or royalties) that con¬flict with material presented in the report.

TABLE OF CONTENTS

EXECUTIVE SUMMARY
Background 1
Methods 2
Data Synthesis 2
Rating the Body of Evidence 2
Peer Review 2
Results 2
Recommendations for Future Research 5
Conclusion 6
Abbreviations Table 6

INTRODUCTION 7
Objective of this Report 7

METHODS
Topic Development 8
Analytic Framework 8
Search Strategy 9
Study Selection 9
Data Abstraction 11
Quality Assessment 11
Data Synthesis 11
Rating the Body of Evidence 11
Peer Review 12

RESULTS
Literature Search 13
Study Characteristics 14
Key Question 1. What are the effects of policy/benefits packages that include vouchers, rebates, premium reductions, or other economic incentives to encourage physical activity through fitness center memberships? 15
Key Question 2. What are the effects of policy/benefits packages that include vouchers, rebates, premium reductions, or other economic incentives to encourage physical activity through fitness center memberships on satisfaction with the health plan and retention of members in the health plan? 17
Key Question 3. Do the effects of policy/benefits packages to encourage physical activity vary by specific characteristics of the package (premium vs. lump sum) or age, sex, and physical illness of participants? 17

SUMMARY AND DISCUSSION 18
Summary of Evidence 18
Implication of Findings 18
Strengths and Limitations 19
Recommendations for Future Research 20
Conclusions 23

REFERENCES	25
APPENDIX A. SEARCH STRATEGIES	27
APPENDIX B. EXCLUDED STUDIES	28
APPENDIX C. DATA ABSTRACTION ELEMENTS	31
APPENDIX D. PEER REVIEW COMMENTS	32
APPENDIX E. GLOSSARY	37

FIGURES

Figure 1.	Analytic framework for assessing effects of health plan-sponsored fitness center benefits	8
Figure 2.	Literature flow diagram	13

TABLES

Table ES-1.	Overview of articles evaluating effects of fitness center membership	3
Table ES-2.	Evidence gaps and future research	6
Table 1.	Summary of inclusion and exclusion criteria	9
Table 2.	Overview of articles evaluating effects of fitness center membership	14
Table 3.	Evidence gaps and future research	20
Table 4.	Comparisons of study designs used to assess effects of health plan-sponsored fitness benefits	22

EXECUTIVE SUMMARY

BACKGROUND

Regular physical activity has many positive health benefits, including protection against chronic disease, improved physical and mental health and cognitive function, and better health-related related quality of life. Moreover, lack of physical activity is associated with higher health care costs and utilization. Many Americans, however, do not get the recommended levels of physical activity. For Veterans, Veterans Affairs (VA) health care users are less likely to meet physical activity recommendations and more likely to be physically inactive compared with Veterans who do not use VA health care. Multiple personal, social, and environmental factors influence participation in physical activity. Providing memberships to fitness centers may be a viable option to increase physical activity and the positive health outcomes associated with such activity. Given that most Americans have access to some form of health insurance, health plan promotion of and coverage for fitness center memberships has the potential to address multiple barriers to physical activity (e.g., cost, access) and extend fitness center access to many Americans.

Our objective in this evidence synthesis was to summarize the results of diverse studies of health plan-sponsored fitness center memberships in an effort to understand how these benefits affect physical activity, clinical outcomes, health care costs and utilization, retention of plan members, and member satisfaction.

Key Question 1. What are the effects of policy/benefits packages that include vouchers, rebates, premium reductions, or other economic incentives to encourage physical activity through fitness center memberships on:

(a) Physical activity participation rates among plan members?
(b) Health outcomes demonstrated to be improved by physical activity (i.e., weight, pain, glucose, blood pressure, health-related quality of life)?
(c) Overall health care costs and health care utilization?

Key Question 2. What are the effects of policy/benefits packages that include vouchers, rebates, premium reductions, or other economic incentives to encourage physical activity through fitness center memberships on satisfaction with the health plan and retention of members in the health plan?

Key Question 3. Do the effects of policy/benefits packages to encourage physical activity vary by specific characteristics of the package (premium vs. lump sum) or age, sex, and physical illness of participants?

METHODS

In consultation with a master librarian, we searched MEDLINE® (via PubMed®), Embase®, and the Cochrane Database of Systematic Reviews for peer-reviewed publications comparing health plan-sponsored strategies to encourage physical activity through fitness center memberships with standard benefit plans from database inception through January 2012. We selected free-text terms to search titles and abstracts as well as validated search terms for both randomized controlled trials and relevant observational studies adapted from the Cochrane Effective Practice & Organization of Care Group search, version 1.9. We limited the search to articles published in the English language involving human subjects 18 years of age and older. An updated search for publications was conducted in May 2012. We also evaluated the bibliographies of included primary studies. As a mechanism to assess the risk of publication bias, we searched www.ClinicalTrials.gov for completed but unpublished studies in July 2012.

DATA SYNTHESIS

We critically analyzed studies to compare their characteristics, methods, and findings to determine the feasibility of completing a quantitative synthesis (i.e., meta-analysis) based on the volume of relevant literature, the completeness of the results reported and the conceptual homogeneity of the studies. As quantitative synthesis was not possible, we analyzed the results qualitatively.

RATING THE BODY OF EVIDENCE

In addition to rating the quality of individual studies, we evaluated the overall strength of evidence (SOE) for each Key Question by assessing the following domains: risk of bias, consistency, directness, precision, strength of association (magnitude of effect), and publication bias. These domains were considered qualitatively, and a summary rating of high, moderate, low, or insufficient SOE was assigned.

PEER REVIEW

A draft version of the report was reviewed by technical experts and clinical leadership. A transcript of their comments can be found in the appendix, which elucidates how each comment was considered in the final report.

RESULTS

We identified 3584 unique citations from a combined search of MEDLINE (via PubMed, n=3560), Embase (n=24), and the Cochrane database (n=0). Manual searching of included study bibliographies and review articles identified 5 additional citations for a total of 3589 citations. After applying inclusion/exclusion criteria, 4 articles (representing 1 unique study) were included in this review. Most studies were excluded because they assessed types of physical activity promotion strategies other than fitness center memberships (e.g., worksite wellness). Our search of www.ClinicalTrials.gov did not suggest publication bias. There were no completed studies that were unpublished. In addition, there were no ongoing studies on this topic.

All articles we identified addressed KQ 1; none addressed KQ 2 or KQ 3 (Table ES-1). The main study was a retrospective cohort study rated fair quality that used administrative and claims data to assess the health care and utilization effects of a health plan-sponsored fitness center membership benefit (known as the Silver Sneakers program) among adults 65 years of age and older who were enrolled in the Group Health Cooperative of Puget Sound Medicare Advantage plan. Two companion articles assessed the effect of distance from the fitness center and history of depression on the uptake of fitness center benefits and frequency of use among participants. One additional companion article assessed the effect of this benefit on health care costs and utilization among health plan members with diabetes. The Silver Sneakers program assessed in all analyses allowed eligible health plan enrollees 65 years of age and older to access selected fitness centers and all activities (e.g., structured conditioning classes) and facilities (e.g., exercise equipment, pool) associated with these fitness centers. The health plan covered the full cost of memberships for each year; there were no additional costs to the member for the fitness center membership.

Table ES-1. Overview of articles evaluating effects of fitness center membership

Reference	Study Details	KQ	Included Outcomes
Main study			
Nguyen et al., 2008	Group Health Cooperative Medicare Advantage enrollees ≥ age 65 Selection dates: Jan 1998–Dec 2003 Participants: 4766 benefit users Matched controls: 9035 benefit nonusers	1a 1c	• Physical activity participation • Health care cost • Health care utilization
Companion articles			
Berke et al., 2006	Group Health Cooperative Medicare Advantage enrollees ≥ age 65 Selection dates: Jan 2002–Dec 2003 Participants: 1728 benefit users Matched controls: 4838 benefit nonusers	1a	Role of distance from fitness center on: • Uptake of benefit • Frequency of use of benefit
Nguyen et al., 2008	Group Health Cooperative Medicare Advantage enrollees ≥ age 65 Selection dates: Jan 1998–Dec 2003 Participants: 4766 benefit users Matched controls: 9035 benefit nonusers	1a	Role of depression history on: • Uptake of benefit • Frequency of use of benefit, risk of participation lapse
Nguyen et al., 2008	Group Health Cooperative Medicare Advantage enrollees ≥ age 65 Selection dates: Jan 1998–Dec 2003 Participants: 618 benefit users with diabetes Matched controls: 1413 benefit nonusers with diabetes	1a 1c	• Physical activity participation • Health care cost • Health care utilization

Key Question 1. What are the effects of policy/benefits packages that include vouchers, rebates, premium reductions, or other economic incentives to encourage physical activity through fitness center memberships on:

(a) Physical activity participation rates among plan members?

(b) Health outcomes demonstrated to be improved by physical activity (i.e., weight, pain, glucose, blood pressure, health-related quality of life)?

(c) Overall health care costs and health care utilization?

KQ 1a: Physical Activity Participation

None of the included articles assessed physical activity as a primary outcome. The only metric of physical activity was the frequency of fitness center visits by participants in the Silver Sneakers program such as that reported in the main study and one companion article. Two additional companion articles assessed the associations between (1) the distance from the fitness center and (2) a history of depression on the uptake and frequency of use of the health plan-sponsored fitness center membership benefit.

In Year 1 of the main study, Silver Sneakers participants averaged 75 visits (median 49; interquartile range [IQR] 11 to 120). In Year 2, the average number of visits declined to 55 (median 12; IQR 0 to 89). While participation dropped in Year 2, 61 percent of participants continued to visit fitness centers. A separate analysis using a subset of members with diabetes from the main study reported similar number of average visits per year (72 visits in Year 1, 49 visits in Year 2).

Two companion articles provided information on other factors associated with uptake and frequency of use. Additional analyses suggest that distance from fitness centers and history of depression influence the uptake of health plan-sponsored fitness center memberships. Enrollment in a fitness center and frequency of use are both associated with distance from gyms. While history of depression is not associated with participation in a fitness center benefit, health plan members with a history of depression made fewer visits and were at greater risk of lapses in their participation compared with nondepressed members.

KQ 1b: Physical Health Outcomes

No identified studies addressed KQ 1b.

KQ 1c: Health Care Costs and Utilization

The main study and one companion article reported the effects of health plan-sponsored fitness center memberships on health care costs and utilization. In adjusted models for Year 1, Nguyen et al. reported that adjusted total health care costs were not different between Silver Sneakers participants and nonparticipants. By the end of Year 2, participants incurred significantly lower total health care costs (-$500; CI -$892 to -$106, p=0.01) likely due to fewer inpatient admissions and lower inpatient care costs compared with controls. There was evidence of a dose-response by average number of health club visits. Compared with participants who attended fitness centers less than one time per week, participants who averaged two to less than three or three or more visits per week over 2 years had lower adjusted health care costs (2 to <3 visits -$1252, p<0.001; ≥ 3 visits -$1309, p=0.001).

In another article, participants in Silver Sneakers with diabetes had lower adjusted total health care costs compared with age- and sex-matched nonparticipants with diabetes after 1 year of enrollment in the fitness center program (-$1633; 95% CI -$2620 to -$646, p=0.001). This cost savings was likely due to fewer hospitalizations and lower adjusted inpatient costs. In Year 2, participants accumulated lower total health care costs, but these savings were not statistically significantly different from diabetic nonparticipants (-$1230; CI -$2494 to $33, p=0.06).

Key Question 2. What are the effects of policy/benefits packages that include vouchers, rebates, premium reductions, or other economic incentives to encourage physical activity through fitness center memberships on satisfaction with the health plan and retention of members in the health plan?

No identified studies addressed KQ 2.

Key Question 3. Do the effects of policy/benefits packages to encourage physical activity vary by specific characteristics of the package (premium vs. lump sum) or age, sex, and physical illness of participants?

No identified studies addressed KQ 3.

RECOMMENDATIONS FOR FUTURE RESEARCH

Surprisingly few studies assessed the impact of health plan-sponsored fitness membership benefits. Existing studies lack diversity in included populations, benefits assessed, outcomes collected, and study designs employed. Across included articles in this review, main limitations were the inability to (1) control for confounding from potential selection bias that could not be accounted for through analysis, (2) rule out concurrent exposures to other sources of physical activity that may have biased results, and (3) measure quality and type of physical activity; the number of visits to the fitness center was the only measure of physical activity. However, a strength of the included studies was that they used existing "real world" administrative and claims data.

A variety of study designs can be employed—each having their own strengths and weaknesses. Researchers must carefully weigh the tradeoffs in costs, feasibility, time, quality of evidence, and generalizability, which differ among the various study design options. We used a structured framework to identify gaps in evidence, classify why these gaps exist, and suggest types of studies to consider in future research (Table ES-2).

Table ES-2. Evidence gaps and future research

Evidence Gap	Reason	Type of Studies to Consider
Patients		
Absence of data for patients other than those ≥ age 65	Insufficient information	• Multisite cluster RCTs • Quasi-experimental studies • Prospective cohort studies
Interventions		
Silver Sneakers program was the only benefit assessed	Insufficient information	• RCTs of head-to-head comparisons of different types of benefit structures • Quasi-experimental studies comparing different types of policy changes that impact benefit structures
Outcomes		
Uncertain effects on: • Physical activity levels • Physical health outcomes • Health care costs and utilization	Insufficient information	• Multisite cluster RCTs • Prospective cohort studies • Nonrandomized trials (pre-post designs) • Nonrandomized controlled before-and-after studies
Uncertain effects on health plan member: • Satisfaction • Retention	Insufficient information	• Multisite cluster RCTs • Prospective or retrospective cohort studies • Nonrandomized controlled before-and-after studies • Qualitative studies

Abbreviation: RCT = randomized controlled trial

CONCLUSION

Health plan-sponsored fitness center memberships have the potential to increase levels of physical activity and, subsequently, improve health and economic outcomes for Veterans. However, few studies have assessed the impact of health plan-sponsored fitness membership benefits. The evidence base for these claims remains weak due to study design limitations, and insufficient due to the paucity of literature. The limited evidence provides support for reductions in health care costs and utilization when comparing health plan members who choose to participate in health plan-sponsored gym memberships with those who do not—but these results may not be generalizable to Veterans and are based on study designs that could be subject to bias. The existing literature provides little insight into other outcomes such as physical activity, physical health outcomes, or health plan member satisfaction or retention. Thus, further evidence is needed on which to base policy recommendations on the merits of providing health plan-sponsored fitness center memberships.

ABBREVIATIONS TABLE

CI	confidence interval
ES	Executive Summary
IQR	interquartile range
KQ	Key Question
RCT	randomized controlled trial
SOE	strength of evidence
VA	Department of Veterans Affairs

EVIDENCE REPORT

INTRODUCTION

Regular physical activity has many positive health benefits, including protection against chronic disease, improved physical and mental health and cognitive function, and better health-related related quality of life.[1-9] Moreover, lack of physical activity is associated with higher health care costs and utilization.[10,11] The current U.S. guidelines recommend that adult Americans (1) engage in at least 150 minutes of moderate-intensity aerobic activity or 75 minutes of vigorous-intensity aerobic activity each week (or an equivalent mix of moderate- and vigorous-intensity aerobic activity) and (2) perform strengthening activities that target all major muscle groups on at least 2 days a week.[12] However, many Americans do not get the recommended levels of physical activity.[13] More Veterans are sufficiently active than non-Veterans. However, Veterans who use Veterans Affairs (VA) health care are more likely to be physically inactive (22.6% vs. 14.9%) and are less likely to meet physical activity recommendations (42.6% vs. 46.7%) compared with Veterans who do not use VA health care.[14]

Multiple personal, social, and environmental factors influence a person's participation in physical activity.[15] Consequently, multiple internal and external barriers to obtaining regular physical activity exist. Internal barriers include a lack of time and motivation, health problems, and emotional difficulties. External barriers involve weather; cultural issues; safety concerns; limited access to facilities, equipment, and transportation; and monetary expenses such as those associated with attending a fitness center. The perceived cost of engaging in physical activity is a significant barrier that increases the likelihood of sedentary behaviors and decreases the likelihood of participation in vigorous physical activity.[16] Thus, reducing the cost of being physically active through providing full or partial memberships to fitness centers may be a viable option to increase physical activity and the positive health outcomes associated with such activity. Given that most Americans (84%) have access to some form of health insurance,[17] health plan promotion of and coverage for fitness center memberships has the potential to address multiple barriers to physical activity (e.g., cost, access) and extend fitness center access to many Americans.

The effects of physical activity on health care utilization and costs, various health outcomes, and general well-being are well established. However, the evidence base on health plan-sponsored benefits—specifically involving fitness center memberships—that support these outcomes has not been synthesized. Therefore, we conducted a systematic review of the current literature to assess the impact of health plan benefits, or policies that promote access to fitness centers, on physical activity levels, health outcomes, overall health care costs and utilization, and satisfaction with and retention in the health plan to inform future Veterans Health Administration (VHA) policy changes.

OBJECTIVE OF THIS REPORT

Our objective in this evidence synthesis was to summarize the results of diverse studies of health plan-sponsored fitness center memberships in an effort to understand how these benefits affect physical activity, clinical outcomes, health care costs and utilization, retention of plan members, and member satisfaction.

METHODS

TOPIC DEVELOPMENT

This review was commissioned by the VA Evidence-based Synthesis Program. The topic was nominated and key questions developed after a refinement process that included a preliminary review of published peer-reviewed literature and consultation with experts, investigators, and key stakeholders. The final key questions (KQs) were:

KQ 1. What are the effects of policy/benefits packages that include vouchers, rebates, premium reductions, or other economic incentives to encourage physical activity through fitness center memberships on:

(a) Physical activity participation rates among plan members?
(b) Health outcomes demonstrated to be improved by physical activity (i.e., weight, pain, glucose, blood pressure, health-related quality of life)?
(c) Overall health care costs and health care utilization?

KQ 2. What are the effects of policy/benefits packages that include vouchers, rebates, premium reductions, or other economic incentives to encourage physical activity through fitness center memberships on satisfaction with the health plan and retention of members in the health plan?

KQ 3. Do the effects of policy/benefits packages to encourage physical activity vary by specific characteristics of the package (premium vs. lump sum) or age, sex, and physical illness of participants?

ANALYTIC FRAMEWORK

The standard protocol used for this review maps to the Preferred Reporting Items for Systematic Reviews and Meta-Analyses (PRISMA) checklist.[18] Our approach was guided by the analytic framework shown in Figure 1.

Figure 1. Analytic framework for assessing effects of health plan-sponsored fitness center benefits

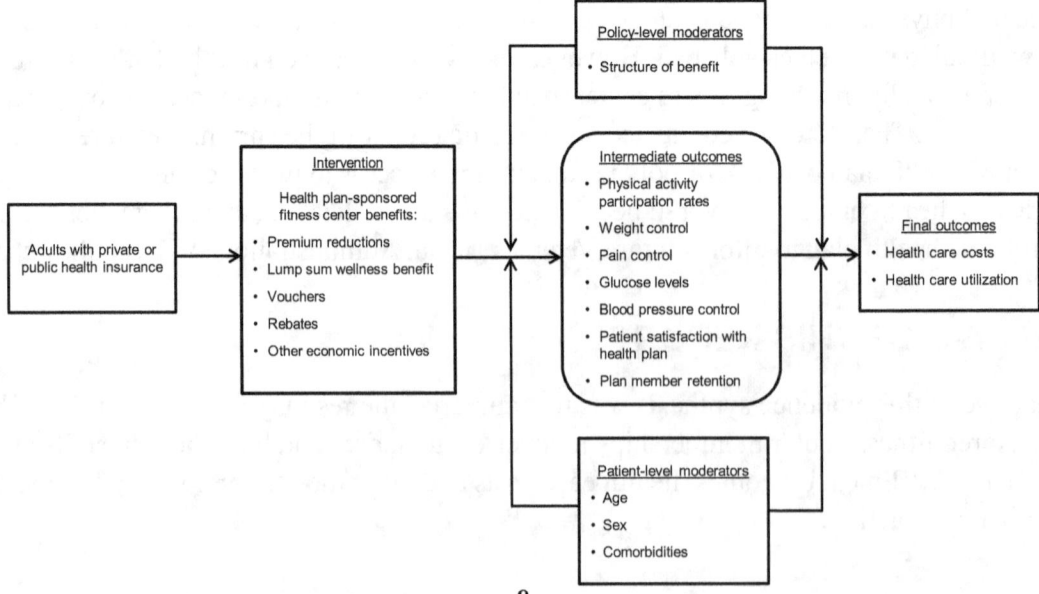

SEARCH STRATEGY

In consultation with a master librarian, we searched MEDLINE® (via PubMed®), Embase®, and the Cochrane Database of Systematic Reviews for peer-reviewed publications comparing health plan-sponsored strategies to encourage physical activity through fitness center memberships with standard benefit plans from database inception through January 2012. We selected free-text terms to search titles and abstracts as well as validated search terms for both randomized controlled trials[19] and relevant observational studies adapted from the Cochrane Effective Practice & Organization of Care Group search, version 1.9. We limited the search to articles published in the English language involving human subjects 18 years of age and older. The full search strategy is provided in Appendix A. An updated search for publications was conducted in May 2012. We also evaluated the bibliographies of included primary studies. All citations were imported into an electronic database, EndNote® Version X5 (Thomson Reuters, Philadelphia, PA) for referencing. As a mechanism to assess the risk of publication bias, we searched www.ClinicalTrials.gov for completed but unpublished studies in July 2012.

STUDY SELECTION

Using prespecified inclusion and exclusion criteria, two reviewers assessed titles and abstracts for relevance to the KQs. Full-text articles identified by either reviewer as potentially relevant were retrieved for further review. Each article retrieved was examined by two other reviewers against the eligibility criteria. Disagreements on inclusion, exclusion, or major reason for exclusion were resolved by discussion or by a third reviewer. The criteria to screen articles for inclusion or exclusion at both the title-and-abstract and full-text screening stages is shown in Table 1. Studies excluded at the full-text review stage are listed with the reasons for exclusion in Appendix B.

Table 1. Summary of inclusion and exclusion criteria

Study characteristic	Inclusion criteria	Exclusion criteria
Population	Adults ≥18 years of age with or without a chronic illness	Studies with populations <18 years of age
Intervention	• Intervention or "exposure" must meet the following definition: Health plan-sponsored strategies (e.g., vouchers, rebates, premium reductions) to encourage physical activity through fitness center memberships If the intervention includes a variety of fitness or exercise-related strategies in addition to facilitating gym memberships, the majority of activities (50% or more) should be like those typically provided through a gym to increase physical activity (e.g., yoga classes, walking clubs, trainer)	Study excluded if exposure meets any of the following criteria: • Studies of health plan-sponsored access to rehabilitation facilities • Studies of access to fitness centers not offered through health plan-sponsored economic incentives • Worksite wellness programs • Interventions that use a wide array of health promotion strategies not typically provided at a fitness center (e.g., health risk assessments, preventive health screenings) if the effects of fitness-related activities are not distinguishable from other components of the intervention

Study characteristic	Inclusion criteria	Exclusion criteria
Comparator	• Standard benefits packages (health plans that do not offer strategies to encourage physical activity through fitness center memberships) • Head-to-head comparisons of different health plan-sponsored programs to encourage physical activity through fitness center memberships	None; study must have a control group
Outcome	KQs 1 and 3: • Physical activity participation rates (e.g., minutes spent being physically active, visits to fitness center) • Weight control (i.e., weight loss or maintenance of current weight) • Pain level using validated measures • Biophysical markers such as laboratory or physiological markers of glucose control or blood pressure • Health-related quality of life • Health care utilization of medical resources (e.g., in-patient admissions, emergency visits, primary care or specialty visits) • Health care costs (prioritizing total health care costs) KQ 2: • Member satisfaction with health plan • Retention of plan members	None
Timing	For longitudinal studies, outcomes must be measured at ≥6 months from start of assessment period	For longitudinal studies, outcomes reported <6 months from start of assessment period
Setting	• Study conducted in North America, Western Europe, Australia, New Zealand[a] • Public or private health plans	Conducted in countries other than those specifically listed as included
Study design[b]	• Original data • Prospective and retrospective observational studies with comparator (sample size ≥100 subjects) • Patient or cluster randomized trials (all sample sizes) • Interrupted time-series designs that have ≥3 measurement points prior to and after the intervention is begun	Cross-sectional studies and other observational study designs not specifically listed as "included" study designs
Publications	• English-language only • Peer-reviewed article	Non-English language publication

[a]Rationale is that medical systems in economically developed countries with sufficient similarities in the system and culture are applicable to U.S. medical care.
[b]Study designs recommended by the Cochrane Effective Practice and Organization of Care Group.
Abbreviation: KQ = Key Question

DATA ABSTRACTION

We designed the data abstraction forms to collect the data required to evaluate the eligibility criteria for inclusion in this review, as well as population characteristics and other data needed for determining outcomes and risk of bias (Appendix C). We paid particular attention to the details of the intervention to assure that it was offered through a health insurance plan as a health benefit and that it was engaged in by the participant at a fitness center. We did not evaluate studies on workplace wellness or health plan access to rehabilitation facilities. One researcher abstracted the data, and a second reviewed the completed abstraction form alongside the original article to check for accuracy and completeness. As with full-text review, disagreements were resolved by discussion or by a third reviewer. We supplemented abstraction of published data by contacting authors for missing information. We contacted one author who replied with additional information about benefits structure and costs.

QUALITY ASSESSMENT

Data necessary for assessing quality and applicability, as described in the Agency for Healthcare Research and Quality (AHRQ) *Methods Guide for Effectiveness and Comparative Effectiveness Reviews*,[20] also were abstracted. Per the AHRQ *Methods Guide*,[20] threats to internal validity of systematic review conclusions based on observational studies were identified through assessment of the body of observational literature as a whole, with an examination of characteristics of individual studies. Study-specific issues that were considered include: potential for selection bias (i.e., degree of similarity between intervention and control patients); performance bias (i.e., differences in care provided to intervention and control patients not related to the study intervention); attribution and detection bias (i.e., whether outcomes were differentially detected between intervention and control groups); and magnitude of reported intervention effects (see the section on "Selecting Observational Studies for Comparing Medical Interventions" in the *Methods Guide*). Using these quality criteria, we assigned a summary quality score (good, fair, poor) to included studies.[20] For each study, two investigators independently assigned a summary quality rating; disagreements were resolved by consensus or by a third investigator as before.

DATA SYNTHESIS

We critically analyzed studies to compare their characteristics, methods, and findings to determine the feasibility of completing a quantitative synthesis (i.e., meta-analysis) based on the volume of relevant literature, the completeness of the results reported and the conceptual homogeneity of the studies. As quantitative synthesis was not possible, we analyzed the results qualitatively.

RATING THE BODY OF EVIDENCE

In addition to rating the quality of individual studies, we evaluated the overall quality of the evidence for each KQ as described in the *Methods Guide*,[20] if feasible. This approach requires assessment of four domains: risk of bias, consistency, directness, and precision. Additional domains considered were strength of association (magnitude of effect) and publication bias. These domains were considered qualitatively, and a summary rating of high, moderate, low, or insufficient strength of evidence was assigned after discussion by two reviewers.

PEER REVIEW

A draft version of the report was reviewed by technical experts and clinical leadership. A transcript of their comments can be found in Appendix D, which elucidates how each comment was considered in the final report.

RESULTS

LITERATURE SEARCH

The flow of articles through the literature search and screening process is illustrated in Figure 2. We identified 3584 unique citations from a combined search of MEDLINE (via PubMed, n=3560), Embase (n=24), and the Cochrane database (n=0). Manual searching of included study bibliographies and review articles identified 5 additional citations for a total of 3589 citations. After applying inclusion/exclusion criteria at the title-and-abstract level, 47 full-text articles were retrieved and screened. Of these, 43 were excluded at the full-text screening stage, leaving 4 articles (representing 1 unique study) for data abstraction. Most studies were excluded at full-text review because they assessed types of physical activity promotion strategies other than fitness center memberships (e.g., worksite wellness) provided through health plan benefits. Our search of www.ClinicalTrials.gov did not suggest publication bias. There were no completed studies that were unpublished. In addition, there were no ongoing studies on this topic.

Figure 2. Literature flow diagram

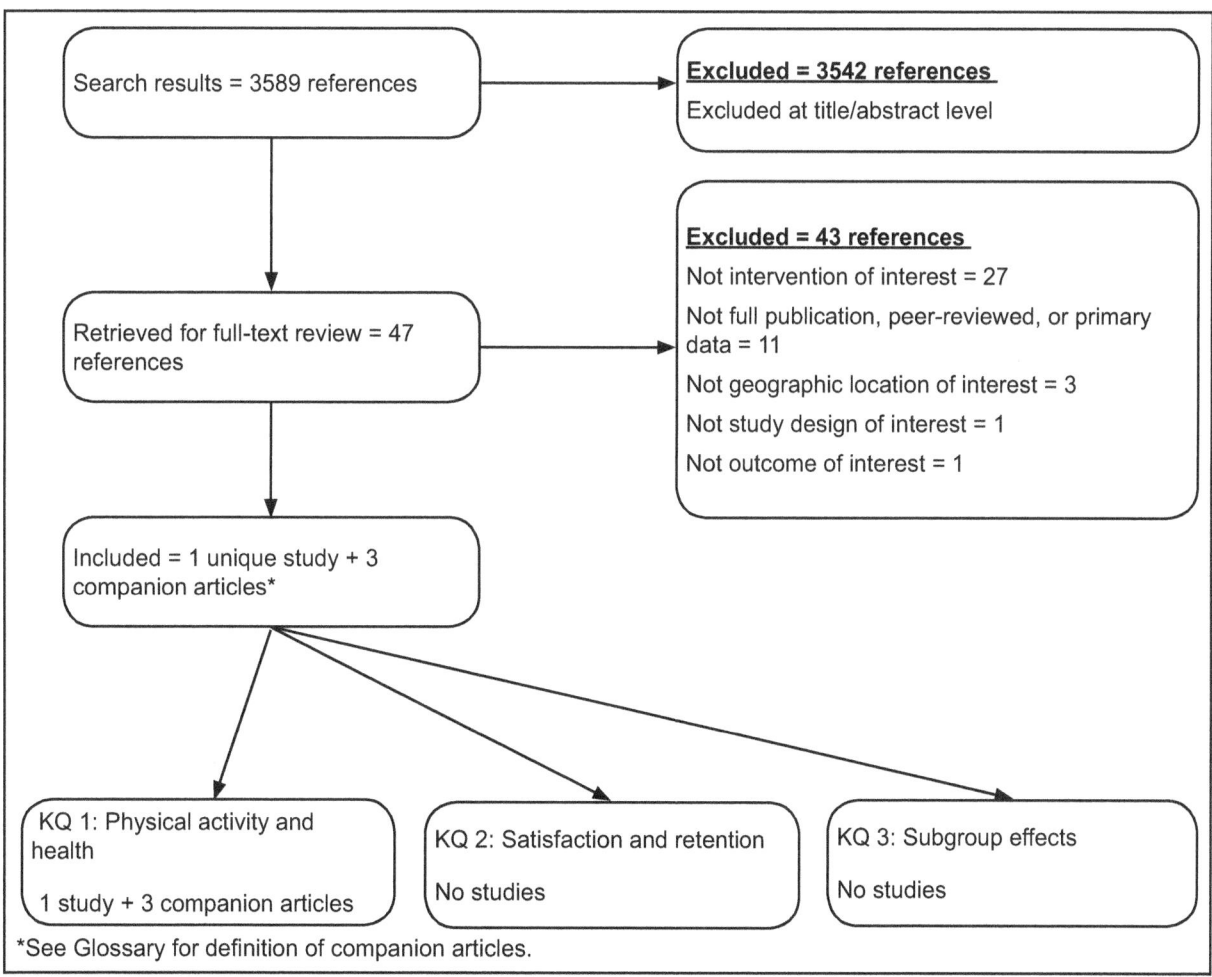

Note: At the request of a peer reviewer, we reconsidered one reference[21] that was initially excluded at the title/abstract level; however, we retained our original conclusion that the reference could not be included based on our inclusion/exclusion criteria.
Abbreviation: KQ = Key Question

STUDY CHARACTERISTICS

Only one main study[22] and three companion articles[23-25] met inclusion criteria for this review (Table 2). All articles we identified addressed KQ 1; none addressed KQ 2 or KQ 3. The main study was a retrospective cohort study rated fair quality that used administrative and claims data to assess the effects of a health plan-sponsored fitness center membership benefit (known as the Silver Sneakers program) on health care costs and utilization among adults 65 years of age and older who were enrolled in the Group Health Cooperative of Puget Sound Medicare Advantage plan. The Group Health Cooperative is a consumer-governed, staff-model, health maintenance organization of more than 500,000 members.

Two companion articles assessed the effect of distance from the fitness center[23] and history of depression[24] on the uptake of fitness center benefits and frequency of use among participants. One additional companion article[25] assessed the effect of this benefit on health care costs and utilization among health plan members with diabetes. All variables used in analyses (e.g., patient demographics, costs) were obtained from health plan administrative data. Relevant results are discussed in detail following the table.

Table 2. Overview of articles evaluating effects of fitness center membership

Reference	Study Details	KQ	Included Outcomes
Main study			
Nguyen et al., 2008[22]	Group Health Cooperative Medicare Advantage enrollees ≥ age 65 Selection dates: Jan 1998–Dec 2003 Participants: 4766 benefit users Matched controls: 9035 benefit nonusers	1a 1c	• Physical activity participation • Health care cost • Health care utilization
Companion articles			
Berke et al., 2006[23]	Group Health Cooperative Medicare Advantage enrollees ≥ age 65 Selection dates: Jan 2002–Dec 2003 Participants: 1728 benefit users Matched controls: 4838 benefit nonusers	1a	Role of distance from fitness center on: • Uptake of benefit • Frequency of use of benefit
Nguyen et al., 2008[24]	Group Health Cooperative Medicare Advantage enrollees ≥ age 65 Selection dates: Jan 1998–Dec 2003 Participants: 4766 benefit users Matched controls: 9035 benefit nonusers	1a	Role of depression history on: • Uptake of benefit • Frequency of use of benefit, risk of participation lapse
Nguyen et al., 2008[25]	Group Health Cooperative Medicare Advantage enrollees ≥ age 65 Selection dates: Jan 1998–Dec 2003 Participants: 618 benefit users with diabetes Matched controls: 1413 benefit nonusers with diabetes	1a 1c	• Physical activity participation • Health care cost • Health care utilization

KEY QUESTION 1. What are the effects of policy/benefits packages that include vouchers, rebates, premium reductions, or other economic incentives to encourage physical activity through fitness center memberships on:

(a) Physical activity participation rates among plan members?

(b) Health outcomes demonstrated to be improved by physical activity (i.e., weight, pain, glucose, blood pressure, health-related quality of life)?

(c) Overall health care costs and health care utilization?

KQ 1a: Physical Activity Participation

None of the included articles assessed physical activity as a primary outcome. The only metric of physical activity was the frequency of fitness center visits by participants in the Silver Sneakers program such as that reported in the main study[22] and one companion article.[25] Two additional companion articles assessed the associations between (1) the distance from the fitness center[23] and (2) a history of depression[24] on the uptake and frequency of use of the health plan-sponsored fitness center membership benefit.

The Silver Sneakers program assessed in all analyses allowed eligible health plan enrollees 65 years of age and older to access selected fitness centers and all activities (e.g., structured conditioning classes) and facilities (e.g., exercise equipment, pool) associated with these fitness centers. Participation in Silver Sneakers was voluntary; participants who opted to enroll contacted their local fitness centers to join. The health plan covered the full cost of memberships for each year; there were no additional costs to the member for the fitness center membership. No other details of the benefit structure or characteristics of selected fitness centers were provided in any of the included articles or through communications with study authors. Visits to the fitness center were documented by swipe cards at participating facilities; average attendance was calculated by dividing all fitness center visits over 2 years by 104 weeks.

In the main study,[22] Nguyen et al. used administrative and claims data from a Medicare Advantage plan administered through a health maintenance organization to assess the effects of the fitness center benefit, Silver Sneakers, on health care costs and utilization among adults 65 years of age and older. In these analyses, Silver Sneakers participants (n = 4766) were compared with up to three age- and sex-matched controls (n = 9035) from the same health plan who did not elect to participate in the health plan-sponsored fitness center benefit. The followup interval was 2 years. Silver Sneakers participants were more likely to be male, have arthritis, use more preventive health services, and have higher total health expenditures at baseline than the age- and sex-matched controls. However, Silver Sneakers participants were less likely to have diabetes or congestive heart failure compared with controls. Main study limitations were the inability to (1) control for confounding from potential selection bias that could not be accounted for through analysis, (2) rule out concurrent exposures to other sources of physical activity that may have biased results, and (3) measure quality and type of physical activity; the number of visits to the fitness center was the only measure of physical activity.

In Year 1, Nguyen et al.[22] reported that the average number of fitness center visits among Silver Sneakers participants was 75 (median 49; interquartile range [IQR] 11 to 120). In Year 2, the average number of visits declined to 55 (median 12; IQR 0 to 89). While participation dropped in Year 2, 61 percent of participants continued to visit fitness centers.

A separate analysis[25] using a subset of members with diabetes (n = 618) from the main study[22] also reported the average number of fitness center visits among participants, which was similar to those reported in the main study. Silver Sneakers participants averaged 72 visits in Year 1 and 49 visits in Year 2.

Two companion articles provided information on other factors associated with uptake and frequency of use. In a separate analysis of 1728 Silver Sneakers participants and 4838 nonparticipants, Berke et al.[23] found that plan members who chose the fitness center benefit lived closer to fitness centers compared with nonparticipants (p = 0.017; adjusted model). The odds of participating in Silver Sneakers decreased by 1.3 percent for every kilometer farther that a plan member lived from a fitness center. Additionally, participants who lived closer to fitness centers used these facilities more frequently than those who lived farther away. Controlling for age, sex, socioeconomic status, distance from center, use of selected preventive services (e.g., cancer screenings, vaccinations), and composite measure of disease burden (i.e., RxRisk[26]), participants made an average of 4.2 visits per month (standard deviation 3.4).

In another analysis using Silver Sneakers participant data, Nguyen et al.[24] assessed the impact of history of depression as identified by International Classification of Diseases (ICD)-9-CM codes on benefit uptake and patterns of use (n = 13,801; 4766 participants and 9035 matched controls). This analysis found that depression in the 12 months before the start of the Silver Sneakers program was not associated with enrollment in the fitness membership benefit (odds ratio 1.03; 95% confidence interval [CI] 0.89 to 1.20, p=0.67; adjusted model). Participants with a depression diagnosis, however, made fewer visits per month to fitness centers compared with participants who were not depressed (range -0.64 to -1.5 visits). Additionally, depressed participants had a 19-percent higher risk of participation lapse (hazard ratio 1.19; 95% CI 1.04 to 1.37, p=0.01; adjusted model) compared with participants who were not depressed at baseline.

KQ 1b: Physical Health Outcomes
No identified studies addressed KQ 1b.

KQ 1c: Health Care Costs and Utilization
The main study[22] and one companion article[25] reported the effects of health plan-sponsored fitness center memberships on health care costs and utilization. In adjusted models for Year 1, Nguyen et al.[22] reported that adjusted total health care costs were not different between Silver Sneakers participants and nonparticipants (+$2; 95% CI -$341 to +$344, p=0.99). However, participants experienced fewer inpatient admissions (-1.0%; CI -2.1% to -0.1%, p=0.5) but made more primary care visits (+0.40; CI 0.27 to 0.53, p<0.001) and specialty care visits (+0.22; CI 0.11 to 0.33, p<0.001) compared with controls. By the end of Year 2, participants incurred significantly lower total health care costs (-$500; CI -$892 to -$106, p=0.01). This decrease was likely due to fewer inpatient admissions (-2.3%; CI -3.3% to -1.2%, p<0.001) and lower inpatient care costs (-$270; CI -$533 to -$6, p=0.05) compared with controls.

Silver Sneakers participants had significantly more primary care visits (+0.26; CI 0.13 to 0.40, p<0.001) and specialty care visits (+0.25; CI 0.14 to 0.36, p<0.001) for Year 2, which resulted in higher costs for those services (primary care: +$80, p<0.001; specialty care: +$37, p=0.14). There was also evidence of a dose-response by average number of health club visits. Compared with participants who attended fitness centers less than one time per week, participants who averaged two to less than three or three or more visits per week over 2 years had lower adjusted health care costs (2 to < 3 visits -$1252, p<0.001; ≥ 3 visits -$1309, p=0.001).

Another article[25] used a subset of participants from the retrospective cohort study.[22] Claims data for 2031 older adults with diabetes were examined to assess the impact of Silver Sneakers on health care utilization and costs among this group. Participants with diabetes (n = 618) were more likely to be male, have lower chronic illness burden, use more preventive health services, have more outpatient visits for arthritis, and make more primary and specialty care visits compared to nonparticipants with diabetes (n =1413). Level of diabetes control, age, and total health care costs at baseline were not significantly different between diabetic participants and nonparticipants.

Participants in Silver Sneakers with diabetes had lower adjusted total health care costs compared with age- and sex-matched nonparticipants with diabetes after 1 year of enrollment in the fitness center program ($1633; 95% CI -$2620 to -$646, p=0.001). This cost savings was likely due to fewer hospitalizations (-3.0%, p=0.07) and lower adjusted inpatient costs (-$1021; CI -$1688 to $367, p=0.002). However, in Year 1 diabetic participants had more primary care visits (0.77; CI 0.34 to 1.2, p<0.001) and primary care costs ($129; CI $32 to $266, p=0.009). In Year 2, participants accumulated lower total health care costs, but these savings were not statistically significantly different from diabetic nonparticipants (-$1230; CI -$2494 to $33, p=0.06).

KEY QUESTION 2. What are the effects of policy/benefits packages that include vouchers, rebates, premium reductions, or other economic incentives to encourage physical activity through fitness center memberships on satisfaction with the health plan and retention of members in the health plan?

No identified studies addressed KQ 2.

KEY QUESTION 3. Do the effects of policy/benefits packages to encourage physical activity vary by specific characteristics of the package (premium vs. lump sum) or age, sex, and physical illness of participants?

No identified studies addressed KQ 3.

SUMMARY AND DISCUSSION

Health plan-sponsored fitness center memberships have the potential to reach many Americans and may be an effective strategy to increase physical activity and its associated health benefits. Surprisingly few studies assessed the impact of health plan-sponsored fitness membership benefits—we identified only one main study and three companion articles that assessed the impact of such benefits. Overall, the data are insufficient to grade the strength of the evidence for health plan-sponsored access to fitness centers through member benefits.

The four included articles provided limited data on rates of physical activity (KQ 1a) and health care costs and utilization (KQ 1c). There were no data on physical health outcomes of interest (i.e., weight, pain, glucose, blood pressure, health related quality of life) (KQ 1b) and none on satisfaction with health plans or retention of plan members (KQ 2). No studies assessed whether effects of health plan benefits varied by characteristics of the participants (KQ 3). Further, only one type of plan was assessed in all analyses; thus, no included studies assessed whether effects of health plan-sponsored fitness center memberships varied by benefit type (KQ 3). Data were of limited applicability; all analyses were conducted exclusively in patients 65 years of age and older and were from one geographic location in the United States.

SUMMARY OF EVIDENCE

None of the included articles assessed physical activity as a primary outcome; the only metric of physical activity provided was descriptive information on frequency of fitness center visits. Overall, health plan members who opted to participate in the health plan-sponsored fitness center memberships made few visits to facilities. In the main study,[22] members averaged 1.44 visits per week in Year 1 and 1.06 visits per week in Year 2. These averages were similar to those reported in a subset of members with diabetes.[25] Additional analyses suggest that distance from fitness centers and history of depression influence the uptake of health plan-sponsored fitness center memberships. Enrollment in a fitness center and frequency of use are both associated with distance from gyms.[23] While history of depression is not associated with participation in a fitness center benefit, health plan members with a history of depression made fewer visits and were at greater risk of lapses in their participation compared with nondepressed members.[24]

We found some limited evidence to support the effects of health plan-sponsored fitness center memberships on health care costs and utilization. While participants in the Silver Sneakers program made more primary and specialty care visits, overall health care costs were significantly lower.[22] These saving were likely due to fewer inpatient admissions. Similar patterns of health care use and costs were seen among health plan members with diabetes.[25]

IMPLICATION OF FINDINGS

The clearest finding of this evidence synthesis is that the existing knowledge base does not provide enough data to make evidence-driven policy recommendations about the health and economic effects of health plan-sponsored fitness center membership benefits. The limited evidence available suggests that, if offered, health plan members will use fitness center memberships. However, internal and external barriers to optimal rates of use of such benefits remain.

Overall, health plan members who opted into the Silver Sneakers program tended to have fewer chronic illnesses. These findings complement a recent study that found health plans offering coverage for fitness center memberships attract and retain enrollees with better self-reported health.[27] Together, these finding suggest that adding fitness center memberships to health plan benefits facilitates favorable selection of healthier enrollees, which in turn may lower health care costs by adding and retaining less costly individuals to the risk pool. However, health systems such as the VA have a higher proportion of individuals with chronic diseases (e.g., obesity, diabetes, arthritis). If the VA is able to engage these populations to use fitness center memberships, the cost savings could be significant, particularly for Veterans whose average weekly attendance is more than 1 visit.[22] The results of the study by Nguyen et al.[25] suggest that there may be an earlier and greater return on investment for populations who are at higher risk. Specifically, diabetic participants in the Silver Sneakers program had greater reductions in total health care expenditures than the general population of participants analyzed in Nguyen et al. (-$1230 vs. $500).[22,25]

Other findings suggest that a participant's distance from the fitness center also plays a role in benefit uptake and, after enrollment, frequency of use.[23] Thus, health insurers who have a large proportion of rural enrollees who travel greater distances to fitness centers may have lower uptake of these benefits. Such health insurers may want to structure fitness center benefits that pay per visit instead of per membership or that automatically discontinue monthly fitness center memberships following lapses in use. This has implications for the VA patient population. Many Veterans travel long distances to access VA facilities. Thus, the VA would have to engage local and community-based facilities (e.g., commercial) closer to Veterans' homes in order to optimize benefit uptake and frequency of use. Also, health plans that have older enrollees with more physical limitations due to chronic health conditions may choose to selectively coordinate with fitness centers that offer appropriate exercise options (e.g., pool-based activities, low-impact aerobics classes). Despite these issues, evidence suggest that health plan members who elect to join fitness center programs incurred lower overall health care costs, even among members with chronic illnesses.[22,25] Health insurers evaluating whether to implement such programs should look for ways to enhance more frequent use of fitness centers over time, such as an attendance requirement for continued access, in the design structure of the benefit.

STRENGTHS AND LIMITATIONS

Our study has a number of strengths, including a protocol-driven review, a comprehensive search, and careful quality assessment. We also allowed inclusion of a wide array of observational and experimental studies and sought to collect both patient-level outcomes (e.g., physical activity levels, biophysical markers) and system-level outcomes (e.g., health care costs, health plan member retention rates). However, limitations to our evidence review exist. The greatest limitation of this review is the lack of relevant studies—and particularly no data relevant to KQ 2 and KQ 3. We limited our search to English-language articles and only included citations from North America, Western Europe, Australia, and New Zealand. We maintained this search limitation because we lacked translation resources and, more importantly, wanted to prioritize studies that were applicable to the U.S. medical system and populations, specifically Veterans. It was the opinion of the investigators and our stakeholders that the resources needed to translate non-English articles had a low potential likelihood of identifying relevant data. To the extent that studies applicable to the United States were published in languages other than English or were conducted outside these countries, we may have failed to include relevant studies. Also, the single included study and its associated companion articles all used retrospective observational designs, which has important implications for the strength of associations explored in these studies. Some key limitations were the limited ability to control for residual confounding due to nonrandomized design, no measure of overall physical activity outside of fitness center visits, and no data on the type and quality of physical activity conducted during fitness center visits. In addition, it is crucial to assess fitness center membership prior to and separate from the rollout of fitness center benefits in order to assess whether the benefit is reaching new or lapsed gym users or supplanting memberships of existing fitness center users. In other words—is the benefit enhancing access for people who are not physically active without the benefit but who would become physically active with the benefit? One strength of the included studies, however, was their use of existing "real world" administrative and claims data.

RECOMMENDATIONS FOR FUTURE RESEARCH

Offering partial or full gym membership discounts is a common practice. For example, according to the Employer Health Benefits 2012 Annual Survey from the Kaiser Family Foundation and Health Research and Educational Trust,[28] 65 percent of all large firms (i.e., 200 or more workers) offer gym membership discounts or onsite exercise facilities—highlighting the need for evaluation and identification of best practices related to this increasingly offered benefit. However, results of our review confirm that the current body of literature is weak and insufficient to identify whether these programs improve outcomes and, if so, what are the best practices associated with implementing them. Thus, additional studies are needed to assess the potential merits, costs, and challenges of health plan-sponsored fitness center benefits in order to better inform VA policy. We used the framework recommended Robinson et al.[29] to identify gaps in evidence and classify why these gaps exist (Table 3).

Table 3. Evidence gaps and future research

Evidence Gap	Reason	Type of Studies to Consider
Patients		
Absence of data for patients other than those ≥ age 65	Insufficient information	• Multisite cluster RCTs • Quasi-experimental studies • Prospective cohort studies
Interventions		
Silver Sneakers program was the only benefit assessed	Insufficient information	• RCTs of head-to-head comparisons of different types of benefit structures • Quasi-experimental studies comparing different types of policy changes that impact benefit structures
Outcomes		
Uncertain effects on: • Physical activity levels • Physical health outcomes • Health care costs and utilization	Insufficient information	• Multisite cluster RCTs • Prospective cohort studies • Nonrandomized trials (pre-post designs) • Nonrandomized controlled before-and-after studies

Evidence Gap	Reason	Type of Studies to Consider
Uncertain effects on health plan member: • Satisfaction • Retention	Insufficient information	• Multisite cluster RCTs • Prospective or retrospective cohort studies • Nonrandomized controlled before-and-after studies • Qualitative studies

Abbreviation: RCT = randomized controlled trial

Potential Study Designs for Future Research

Existing studies lack diversity in included populations, benefits assessed, outcomes collected, and study designs employed. There are numerous possibilities regarding future research in this area. In particular, a variety of study designs can be employed—each having their own strengths and weaknesses. Three broad types of possible study designs and specific examples are introduced in Table 4, including (1) experimental (e.g., cluster randomized controlled trial), (2) quasi-experimental (e.g., interrupted time series design), and (3) observational (e.g., prospective cohort study, retrospective cohort study using administrative data).

A cluster randomized controlled trial is a form of randomized controlled trial where groups of subjects or sites (e.g., VA medical centers) are the unit of randomization to treatment or control rather than individual participants. An interrupted time series design involves multiple measurements prior to and following an event (e.g., policy change to add fitness center membership benefits), which allows for evaluation of temporal trends but does not include randomization to study conditions. In an observational prospective cohort study, a defined group of individuals is followed over time before outcomes and exposures are measured. Retrospective cohort studies examine past exposures and outcomes. Table 4 gives an overview of the major strengths and limitations of these selected study design alternatives tailored to future research on health plan-sponsored fitness center memberships. We considered a variety of domains such as level of control over benefit structure, measurement/assessment, internal validity, generalizability, and feasibility (e.g., time, cost).

Table 4. Comparisons of study designs used to assess effects of health plan-sponsored fitness benefits

Study Designs	Major Strengths	Major Limitations
Cluster randomized controlled trial	• Randomization to treatment (i.e., the fitness benefit) or control minimizes the influence of unaccounted, unmeasured factors (i.e., confounding variables) and reduces selection bias. • Substantial control exists over measurement, such as included measures, as well as length of followup and timing. • There is greater strength of evidence and confidence in results/causality. • There is the greatest level of control over structure of the intervention (i.e., benefit). • There is the possibility of comparing different benefit structures using multiple active comparators (i.e., comparative effectiveness trials).	• Threats to validity are still possible if randomization is not successful; results also may be undermined if significant and/or differential dropouts occur. • Design is potentially time-consuming, with a longer lag time in generating findings compared to retrospective cohort studies using existing administrative data. • Design has potentially higher costs than retrospective cohort studies using existing administrative data. • External validity/generalizability is potentially limited if there is a highly selected population, setting, and tightly controlled implementation with resources/staff not available in "real world" settings. • Design may pose a measurement burden for participants.
Interrupted time series design	• This design allows assessment of temporal trends in variables of interest before and after the event (i.e., policy change to include fitness center memberships). • There is potentially lower cost than RCTs and prospective designs if using existing data sources.	• This design has a lack of control over unaccounted, unmeasured factors (i.e., confounding variables). • Design is potentially less feasible; it would need to identify an event and have access to relevant data before and after a policy change. • Design may require a large sample size. • There is no control over structure of benefit unless policymakers consult with researcher.
Prospective cohort study	• Substantial control exists over measurement, such as measure diversity (number and type), as well as length of followup and timing. • There is greater "real-world" applicability compared to tightly controlled randomized trials. • There is greater strength of evidence than with other observational designs such as case-control and retrospective cohort designs because the sequence of event can be assessed.	• Time and cost investment is likely substantial because of the need for a large sample size and multiple assessments. • There is a significant measurement burden for participants. • This design is potentially less feasible and must identify the setting prior to benefit and enrollment, which may pose a significant logistical barrier. • There is a greater risk of bias, lower quality, and lower strength of evidence compared to RCTs. • There is no control over the structure of benefit.
Retrospective cohort study using administrative data	• This design is convenient if datasets are available and accessible (e.g., claims data). • Time and costs required are potentially less than other designs. • This design uses a similar method to existing studies, making it possible to confirm/replicate prior findings.	• Design is limited by the information available and existing variables (e.g., type, quality, timing, followup). • Relevant data must be available and affordable; a large sample size is necessary to create a cohort of interest and define an adequate control group. • Compared to other designs, risk of bias is highest and quality and strength of evidence are lowest. • There is no control over the structure of benefit.

Abbreviation: RCT = randomized controlled trial

When weighing which study designs to use, researchers should always start with what is the best design to answer the research question at hand. However, researchers must also carefully weigh the tradeoffs in costs, feasibility, time, quality of evidence, and generalizability, which differ among the various study design options. Previous research on health plan-sponsored access to fitness memberships has exclusively used retrospective observational designs. Compared with prospective or experimental designs, retrospective observational designs allow for rapid generation of findings if existing data can be used. However, they offer the lowest strength of evidence when compared with the other designs described above and do not allow for control over the benefit structure. Moreover, retrospective observational designs may offer only limited information on complex behaviors like physical activity. The existing literature is limited in this regard and only provides descriptive information on the number of gym visits. Future studies should assess the quality of the physical activity (e.g., moderate vs. vigorous) and the time spent engaging in the activity.

Prospective cohort and quasi-experimental designs, such as interrupted time series designs, provide greater strength of evidence through establishing temporality of events compared with retrospective designs, as well as offering control over the type and quality of measures collected. These designs also come at higher costs, are more time consuming, may pose significant measurement burden on participants, and are impractical for rare events such as shifts in policies. In addition, these designs do not allow for control over the structure of the benefits. Also for interrupted time series designs, it can be difficult to disentangle the effects of the benefit from natural temporal trends without establishing a contemporaneous control group, and use of existing datasets may limit the quality and type of variables assessed.

When assessing the impact of providing memberships to fitness centers through health plan-sponsored benefits, RCTs offer the greatest strength of evidence. These designs also allow for control over the intervention tested (i.e., the benefit structure). Moreover, randomized designs can allow for direct comparisons of different benefit structures through comparative effectiveness trials (head-to-head comparisons). Also, RCTs can allow testing of different incentive strategies (e.g., cash rewards, premium discounts, loss of benefit based on attendance) to encourage continued use of fitness centers. Measurement of complex outcomes like physical activity can be built into the design of trials through the use of objective and automatic physical activity monitoring (e.g., pedometers with wireless data upload). However, randomized trials also tend to be costly and time consuming. In addition, the evidence generated may have limited generalizability if the study was conducted in a tightly controlled research environment with highly selected populations. Efficiencies can be built into theses design such as using cluster randomized designs and using existing data sources such as VA electronic medical records.

CONCLUSIONS

Health plan-sponsored fitness center memberships have the potential to increase levels of physical activity and, subsequently, improve health and economic outcomes for Veterans. However, few studies have assessed the impact of health plan-sponsored fitness membership benefits. The evidence base for these claims remains weak due to study design limitations, and insufficient due to the paucity of literature. The limited evidence provides support for reductions in health care costs and utilization when comparing health plan members who choose to participate in health plan-sponsored gym memberships with those who do not—but these results may not be generalizable to Veterans and are based on study designs that could be subject to bias. The existing literature provides little insight into other outcomes such as physical activity, physical health outcomes, or health plan member satisfaction or retention. Thus, further evidence is needed on which to base policy recommendations on the merits of providing health plan-sponsored fitness center memberships.

REFERENCES

1. Bauman AE. Updating the evidence that physical activity is good for health: an epidemiological review 2000-2003. *J Sci Med Sport*. 2004;7(1 Suppl):6-19.

2. Vogel T, Brechat PH, Lepretre PM, et al. Health benefits of physical activity in older patients: a review. *Int J Clin Pract*. 2009;63(2):303-20.

3. Tseng CN, Gau BS, Lou MF. The effectiveness of exercise on improving cognitive function in older people: a systematic review. *J Nurs Res*. 2011;19(2):119-31.

4. Bize R, Johnson JA, Plotnikoff RC. Physical activity level and health-related quality of life in the general adult population: a systematic review. *Prev Med*. 2007;45(6):401-15.

5. Glenister D. Exercise and mental health: a review. *J R Soc Health*. 1996;116(1):7-13.

6. Gerber M, Puhse U. Review article: do exercise and fitness protect against stress-induced health complaints? A review of the literature. *Scand J Public Health*. 2009;37(8):801-19.

7. Penedo FJ, Dahn JR. Exercise and well-being: a review of mental and physical health benefits associated with physical activity. *Curr Opin Psychiatry*. 2005;18(2):189-93.

8. Bucksch J, Schlicht W. Health-enhancing physical activity and the preventionof chronic diseases--an epidemiological review. *Soz Praventivmed*. 2006;51(5):281-301.

9. Taylor AH, Cable NT, Faulkner G, et al. Physical activity and older adults: a review of health benefits and the effectiveness of interventions. *J Sports Sci*. 2004;22(8):703-25.

10. Franklin BA. Physical activity to combat chronic diseases and escalating health care costs: the unfilled prescription. *Curr Sports Med Rep*. 2008;7(3):122-5.

11. Colditz GA. Economic costs of obesity and inactivity. *Med Sci Sports Exerc*. 1999;31(11 Suppl):S663-7.

12. Department of Health and Human Services. Centers for Disease Control and Prevention. 2008 Physical Activity Guidelines for Americans. Available at: http://www.cdc.gov/physicalactivity/everyone/guidelines/adults.html. Accessed August 1, 2012.

13. Department of Health and Human Services. Centers for Disease Control and Prevention. 2007 U.S. Physical Activity Statistics. Available at: http://apps.nccd.cdc.gov/PASurveillance/StateSumResultV.asp?CI=&Year=2007&State=0#data Accessed August 1, 2012.

14. Littman AJ, Forsberg CW, Koepsell TD. Physical activity in a national sample of veterans. *Med Sci Sports Exerc*. 2009;41(5):1006-13.

15. Cerin E, Leslie E, Sugiyama T, et al. Perceived barriers to leisure-time physical activity in adults: an ecological perspective. *J Phys Act Health*. 2010;7(4):451-9.

16. Salmon J, Owen N, Crawford D, et al. Physical activity and sedentary behavior: a population-based study of barriers, enjoyment, and preference. *Health Psychol*. 2003;22(2):178-88.

17. U.S. Census Bureau. Health Insurance Highlights 2010. Available at: http://www.census.gov/hhes/www/hlthins/data/incpovhlth/2010/highlights.html. Accessed August 1, 2012.

18. Moher D, Liberati A, Tetzlaff J, et al. Preferred reporting items for systematic reviews and meta-analyses: the PRISMA statement. *J Clin Epidemiol*. 2009;62(10):1006-12.

19. Wilczynski NL, McKibbon KA, Haynes RB. Response to Glanville et al.: How to identify randomized controlled trials in MEDLINE: ten years on. *J Med Libr Assoc*. 2007;95(2):117-8; author reply 119-20.

20. Agency for Healthcare Research and Quality. Methods Guide for Effectiveness and Comparative Effectiveness Reviews. Rockville, MD: Agency for Healthcare Research and Quality. Available at: http://www.effectivehealthcare.ahrq.gov/search-for-guides-reviews-and-reports/?pageaction=displayproduct&mp=1&productID=318. Accessed August 1, 2012.

21. Fody-Urias BM, Fillit H, Hill J. The effect of a fitness program on health status and health care consumption in Medicare MCOs. *Manag Care Interface*. 2001;14(9):58-64.

22. Nguyen HQ, Ackermann RT, Maciejewski M, et al. Managed-Medicare health club benefit and reduced health care costs among older adults. *Prev Chronic Dis*. 2008;5(1):A14.

23. Berke EM, Ackermann RT, Lin EH, et al. Distance as a barrier to using a fitness-program benefit for managed medicare enrollees. *J Aging Phys Act*. 2006;14(3):313-323.

24. Nguyen HQ, Koepsell T, Unutzer J, et al. Depression and use of a health plan-sponsored physical activity program by older adults. *Am J Prev Med*. 2008;35(2):111-7.

25. Nguyen HQ, Maciejewski ML, Gao S, et al. Health care use and costs associated with use of a health club membership benefit in older adults with diabetes. *Diabetes Care*. 2008;31(8):1562-7.

26. Putnam KG, Buist DS, Fishman P, et al. Chronic disease score as a predictor of hospitalization. *Epidemiology*. 2002;13(3):340-6.

27. Cooper AL, Trivedi AN. Fitness memberships and favorable selection in Medicare Advantage plans. *N Engl J Med*. 2012;366(2):150-7.

28. The Kaiser Family Foundation and Health Research Educational Trust. Employer Health Benefits 2012 Annual Survey. Available at: http://ehbs.kff.org/. Accessed September 27, 2012.

29. Robinson KA, Saldanha IJ, Mckoy NA. Frameworks for Determining Research Gaps During Systematic Reviews. Methods Future Research Needs Report No. 2. (Prepared by the Johns Hopkins University Evidence-based Practice Center under Contract No. HHSA 290-2007-10061-I.) AHRQ Publication No. 11-EHC043-EF. Rockville, MD: Agency for Healthcare Research and Quality. June 2011. Available at: www.effectivehealthcare.ahrq.gov/reports/final.cfm. Accessed May 22, 2012.

APPENDIX A. SEARCH STRATEGIES

Search strategy for RCTs and observational studies (PubMed, May 2012)

Step	Category	Terms	Results
1	Fitness center terms	"Health Promotion/economics"[Mesh]) OR "Insurance Benefits"[Mesh]) OR "Insurance Claim Review"[Mesh]) OR "Insurance, Health"[Mesh]	116141
2		"Fitness Centers"[Mesh]	281
3		(fitness[tiab] OR health[tiab] OR exercise[tiab] OR recreation[tiab] OR recreational[tiab] OR sports[tiab] OR aquatic[tiab]) AND (club[tiab] OR clubs[tiab] OR membership[tiab] OR memberships[tiab] OR center[tiab] OR centers[tiab] OR program[tiab] OR programs[tiab])	151793
4		gym[tiab] OR gyms[tiab] OR ymca[tiab] OR "community based"[tiab]	29217
5		#1 AND (#2 OR #3 OR #4)	8751
6	Study design terms	(randomized controlled trial[pt] OR controlled clinical trial[pt] OR randomized[tiab] OR randomised[tiab] OR randomization[tiab] OR randomisation[tiab] OR placebo[tiab] OR drug therapy[sh] OR randomly[tiab] OR trial[tiab] OR groups[tiab] OR Clinical trial[pt] OR "clinical trial"[tw] OR "clinical trials"[tw] OR "evaluation studies"[Publication Type] OR "evaluation studies as topic"[MeSH Terms] OR "evaluation study"[tw] OR evaluation studies[tw] OR "intervention studies"[MeSH Terms] OR "intervention study"[tw] OR "intervention studies"[tw] OR "case-control studies"[MeSH Terms] OR "case-control"[tw] OR "cohort studies"[MeSH Terms] OR cohort[tw] OR "longitudinal studies"[MeSH Terms] OR "longitudinal"[tw] OR longitudinally[tw] OR "prospective"[tw] OR prospectively[tw] OR "retrospective studies"[MeSH Terms] OR "retrospective"[tw] OR "follow up"[tw] OR "comparative study"[Publication Type] OR "comparative study"[tw] OR systematic[subset] OR "meta-analysis"[Publication Type] OR "meta-analysis as topic"[MeSH Terms] OR "meta-analysis"[tw] OR "meta-analyses"[tw]) NOT (Editorial[ptyp] OR Letter[ptyp] OR Case Reports[ptyp] OR Comment[ptyp]) NOT (animals[mh] NOT humans[mh])	4383508
7		#5 AND #6	3601

APPENDIX B. EXCLUDED STUDIES

All articles listed below were reviewed in their full-text version and excluded for the reason indicated. An alphabetical reference list follows the table.

Excluded studies with reasons

Reference	Not full publication, peer-reviewed, or primary data	Not English language	Not geographic location of interest	Not intervention of interest	Not study design of interest	Not outcome of interest
Abildso, 2010					X	
Ackermann, 2003				X		
Ackermann, 2008				X		
Anderson, 2001	X					
Anonymous, 2008	X					
Arlton, 1986	X					
Atherly, 2011				X		
Bartlett-Prescott, 2005				X		
Bertera, 1990	X					
Breuleux, 1993				X		
Burnes, 1995	X					
Compton, 2006				X		
Cooper, 2012						X
Cox, 1981				X		
Deitz, 2005				X		
Fielding, 1982	X					
Foote, 2006	X					
Gillman, 2001				X		
Goetzel, 2001	X					
Goetzel, 1998				X		
Haltiwanger, 2007	X					
Hochart, 2011				X		
Kulesher, 2005	X					
Lambert, 2009			X			
Mayer, 2010				X		
Nguyen, 2007				X		
Orme-Johnson, 1997				X		
Ozminkowski, 2001	X					
Ozminkowski, 2006				X		
Ozminkowski, 2002				X		
Patel, 2011			X			
Patel, 2010			X			
Pelletier, 2005				X		
Pronk, 2002				X		
Serxner, 2001				X		
Shephard, 1982				X		
Shephard, 1983				X		
Shephard, 1982				X		
Spencer, 1996				X		
Spilman, 1986				X		
Stevens, 1998				X		
Terry, 1991				X		
Wylie-Rosett, 2001				X		

Note: At the request of a peer reviewer, we reconsidered one reference[21] that was initially excluded at the title/abstract level; however, we retained our original conclusion that the reference could not be included based on our inclusion/exclusion criteria.

LIST OF EXCLUDED STUDIES

Agency for Healthcare Research and Quality. Group Abildso CG, Zizzi SJ, Reger-Nash B. Evaluating an insurance-sponsored weight management program with the RE-AIM Model, West Virginia, 2004-2008. *Prev Chronic Dis*. 2010;7(3):A46.

Ackermann RT, Cheadle A, Sandhu N, et al. Community exercise program use and changes in healthcare costs for older adults. *Am J Prev Med*. 2003;25(3):232-7.

Ackermann RT, Williams B, Nguyen HQ, et al. Healthcare cost differences with participation in a community-based group physical activity benefit for medicare managed care health plan members. *J Am Geriatr Soc*. 2008;56(8):1459-65.

Anderson DR, Serxner SA, Gold DB. Conceptual framework, critical questions, and practical challenges in conducting research on the financial impact of worksite health promotion. *Am J Health Promot*. 2001;15(5):281-8.

Anonymous. Active seniors decrease health costs: Silver Sneakers study shows significant benefits in year two. *Dis Manag Advis*. 2008;14(5):7-9, 1.

Arlton D. A paying health promotion clinic: combining client services and student learning. *J Allied Health*. 1986;15(1):3-10.

Atherly A, Thorpe KE. Analysis of the treatment effect of Healthways' Medicare Health Support Phase 1 Pilot on Medicare costs. *Popul Health Manag*. 2011;14 Suppl 1:S23-8.

Bartlett-Prescott JD, Klesges LM, Kritchevsky SB. Health promotion referrals in an urban clinic: removing financial barriers influences physician but not patient behavior. *Am J Health Promot*. 2005;19(5):376-82.

Bertera RL. The effects of workplace health promotion on absenteeism and employment costs in a large industrial population. *Am J Public Health*. 1990;80(9):1101-5.

Breuleux C, Heck SK, Hollenback J, et al. Preliminary comparison of medical care costs between fitness center members and nonmembers. *Am J Health Promot*. 1993;7(6):405-7.

Burnes H. Personal health improvement program. *HMO Pract*. 1995;9(2):59-60.

Compton MT, Weiss PS, Phillips VL, et al. Determinants of health plan membership among patients in routine U.S. psychiatric practice. *Community Ment Health J*. 2006;42(2):197-204.

Cooper AL, Trivedi AN. Fitness memberships and favorable selection in Medicare Advantage plans. *N Engl J Med*. 2012;366(2):150-7.

Cox M, Shephard RJ, Corey P. Influence of an employee fitness programme upon fitness, productivity and absenteeism. *Ergonomics*. 1981;24(10):795-806.

Deitz D, Cook R, Hersch R. Workplace health promotion and utilization of health services: follow-up data findings. *J Behav Health Serv Res*. 2005;32(3):306-19.

Fielding JE. Effectiveness of employee health improvement programs. *J Occup Med*. 1982;24(11):907-16.

Foote SM. Medicare health support: reinventing chronic care. *Am Heart Hosp J*. 2006;4(1):39-42.

Gillman MW, Pinto BM, Tennstedt S, et al. Relationships of physical activity with dietary behaviors among adults. *Prev Med*. 2001;32(3):295-301.

Goetzel RZ. The financial impact of health promotion and disease prevention programs--why is it so hard to prove value? *Am J Health Promot*. 2001;15(5):277-80.

Goetzel RZ, Dunn RL, Ozminkowski RJ, et al. Differences between descriptive and multivariate estimates of the impact of Chevron Corporation's Health Quest Program on medical expenditures. *J Occup Environ Med*. 1998;40(6):538-45.

Haltiwanger R. Medicare health support program: better quality of life for chronically ill seniors. *Tenn Med*. 2007;100(7):33.

Hochart C, Lang M. Impact of a comprehensive worksite wellness program on health risk, utilization, and health care costs. *Popul Health Manag*. 2011;14(3):111-6.

Kulesher RR. Medicare-the development of publicly financed health insurance: Medicare's impact on the nation's health care system. *Health Care Manag (Frederick)*. 2005;24(4):320-9.

Lambert EV, da Silva R, Fatti L, et al. Fitness-related activities and medical claims related to hospital admissions - South Africa, 2006. *Prev Chronic Dis*. 2009;6(4):A120.

Mayer C, Williams B, Wagner EH, et al. Health care costs and participation in a community-based health promotion program for older adults. *Prev Chronic Dis*. 2010;7(2):A38.

Nguyen HQ, Ackermann RT, Berke EM, et al. Impact of a managed-Medicare physical activity benefit on health care utilization and costs in older adults with diabetes. *Diabetes Care*. 2007;30(1):43-8.

Orme-Johnson DW, Herron RE. An innovative approach to reducing medical care utilization and expenditures. *Am J Manag Care*. 1997;3(1):135-44.

Ozminkowski RJ, Goetzel RZ. Getting closer to the truth: overcoming research challenges when estimating the financial impact of worksite health promotion programs. *Am J Health Promot*. 2001;15(5):289-95.

Ozminkowski RJ, Goetzel RZ, Wang F, et al. The savings gained from participation in health promotion programs for Medicare beneficiaries. *J Occup Environ Med*. 2006;48(11):1125-32.

Ozminkowski RJ, Ling D, Goetzel RZ, et al. Long-term impact of Johnson & Johnson's Health & Wellness Program on health care utilization and expenditures. *J Occup Environ Med*. 2002;44(1):21-9.

Patel D, Lambert EV, da Silva R, et al. Participation in fitness-related activities of an incentive-based health promotion program and hospital costs: a retrospective longitudinal study. *Am J Health Promot*. 2011;25(5):341-8.

Patel DN, Lambert EV, da Silva R, et al. The association between medical costs and participation in the vitality health promotion program among 948,974 members of a South African health insurance company. *Am J Health Promot*. 2010;24(3):199-204.

Pelletier KR. A review and analysis of the clinical and cost-effectiveness studies of comprehensive health promotion and disease management programs at the worksite: update VI 2000-2004. *J Occup Environ Med*. 2005;47(10):1051-8.

Pronk NP, Boucher JL, Gehling E, et al. A platform for population-based weight management: description of a health plan-based integrated systems approach. *Am J Manag Care*. 2002;8(10):847-57.

Serxner S, Gold D, Anderson D, et al. The impact of a worksite health promotion program on short-term disability usage. *J Occup Environ Med*. 2001;43(1):25-9.

Shephard RJ, Corey P, Renzland P, et al. The influence of an employee fitness and lifestyle modification program upon medical care costs. *Can J Public Health*. 1982;73(4):259-63.

Shephard RJ, Corey P, Renzland P, et al. The impact of changes in fitness and lifestyle upon health care utilization. *Can J Public Health*. 1983;74(1):51-4.

Shephard RJ, Corey P, Renzland P, et al. Fitness program reduces health care costs. *Dimens Health Serv*. 1982;59(1):14-5.

Spencer LS, Pratt DS, Hausman A. Using health benefits as an incentive to change employee health risks: preliminary program results. *Empl Benefits J*. 1996;21(2):26-9, 36.

Spilman MA, Goetz A, Schultz J, et al. Effects of a corporate health promotion program. *J Occup Med*. 1986;28(4):285-9.

Stevens W, Hillsdon M, Thorogood M, et al. Cost-effectiveness of a primary care based physical activity intervention in 45-74 year old men and women: a randomised controlled trial. *Br J Sports Med*. 1998;32(3):236-41.

Terry PE, Pheley AM. Health risks and educational interests in an HMO. *HMO Pract*. 1991;5(1):3-6.

Wylie-Rosett J, Swencionis C, Ginsberg M, et al. Computerized weight loss intervention optimizes staff time: the clinical and cost results of a controlled clinical trial conducted in a managed care setting. *J Am Diet Assoc*. 2001;101(10):1155-62; quiz 1163-4.

APPENDIX C. DATA ABSTRACTION ELEMENTS

Study Characteristics:
- Study design
- Study dates
- Study setting
- Geographical location
- Funding source
- Subject selection/enrollment in study
- Source of comparator population and comparator strategy
- Patient eligibility criteria for study matching characteristics

Population Characteristics:
- Number of subjects
- Gender
- Race
- Age
- Education
- Baseline physical activity level
- Smoking status
- Weight
- HbA1c (%)
- Lipids (total cholesterol, LDL, HDL)
- Blood pressure (systolic, diastolic)
- Other relevant comorbid conditions and baseline characteristics (e.g., comorbidities, preventive services index, health care use, health care costs, distance to fitness facility, income)

Intervention Components:
- Components of benefit
- Structure of benefit (e.g., vouchers, rebates, premium reductions)
- Payment structure
- Type of fitness centers available through benefit

Outcome Components:
- Physical activity participation rates
- Weight control
- Pain level using validated measures
- Biophysical markers
  - Glucose control
  - Blood pressure control
- Health-related quality of life
- Health care utilization of medical resources
- Health care costs
- Patient satisfaction with health plan
- Retention of plan members

APPENDIX D. PEER REVIEW COMMENTS

Reviewer	Comment	Response
Question 1: Are the objectives, scope, and methods for this review clearly described?		
1	Yes. The scope is clear but the aims are worded as if the focus is on whether benefit packages that include incentives for fitness center use increase physical activity. Clearly the scope is broader than this, as evidenced by the conceptual model and the sub aims of key question #1. There are a multitude of health benefit designs that involve incentives. The goal is more generally to improve health, reduce costs, and to meet a market demand (i.e. a more common reason employer health executives report including incentives is that they are "part of the plan"; in other words, they can't get by designing a health benefit package any longer that leaves health and wellness benefits out of the package – there is a demand among purchasers). The review searched for effects beyond physical activity. I would recommend rewording the key questions to reflect the interest in whether benefits result in improved health when they include incentives to use a fitness facility. This frames the focus on broader metrics of improved health but still defines the focus on fitness facilities, as opposed to the multitude of other health/wellness programs and incentives in the marketplace today.

I have to keep reminding myself that the focus is really very specifically on incentives to encourage fitness center use. The "effects" are broader than physical activity (e.g. participation, downstream effects of PA, and cost/utilization). Consider: What are the effects of policy/benefits packages that include vouchers, rebates, premium reductions, or other economic incentives to improve health specifically through encouraging the use of fitness centers. | Thank you. We agree that the scope is beyond physical activity. The Key Questions, however, were created in collaboration with, and approved by, the technical expert partners and stakeholders. Therefore, we cannot modify them at this time for the report. |
2	Yes, and no comments from reviewer 2.	Thank you.
3	Yes, and no comments from reviewer 3.	Thank you.
4	Yes. Clear delineation of purpose and KQs, scope is defined with clear inclusion criteria and exclusion criteria, and the methods follow clearly outlined systematic review processes.	Thank you.
Question 2: Is there any indication of bias in our synthesis of the evidence?		
1	No. I do think that there are likely a large number of "program evaluations" that have been conducted by employers or health plans to ascertain net costs of such a benefit. To the extent that these evaluations are absent from the literature, it likely implies that they were negative studies or of poor quality.	Thank you. We agree, and our focus was on peer-reviewed, published literature.
2	No, and no comments from reviewer 2.	Thank you.
3	No, and no comments from reviewer 3.	Thank you.
4	No. Transparency in logic makes the results of the logic flow consistent with the findings presented	Thank you.
Question 3: Are there any published or unpublished studies that we may have overlooked?		
1	No. I do not know of any. There was a study by Fody-Urias about 10 years ago that looked at SS, but I believe it was uncontrolled and likely of limited methodologic rigor.	Thank you. This study was excluded during citation screening but marked for background. Although this paper did look at Silver Sneakers, the study design was not one of interest because there was no control group.

Reviewer	Comment	Response
2	It would have been useful and relevant to look at or contrast the literature of **employer sponsored programs** to encourage PA through fitness center memberships. Whether an employer sponsored vs healthplan sponsored seems like a trivial distinction in terms of potential outcomes and mechanism related to effectiveness.	Thank you. Employer-sponsored programs were not in the scope of the project. This project was focused on the VA context (i.e., health plan members as opposed to employees).
3	No, and no comments from reviewer 3	Thank you.
4	No. The search was in-depth and appears to have included the correct type of studies. Personally, I am also not aware of any other research studies that have been reported in this area.	Thank you.
Question 4: Please write additional suggestions or comments below. If applicable, please indicate the page and line numbers from the draft report.		
1	There are a few missed opportunities to frame the discussion for consumption by both the VA and the research community. I have highlighted three of these in comment boxes on the draft. There is also a fourth, related to behavioral economics, which is also discussed below. First, the authors should review and reference the Kaiser Family Foundation annual employer survey. In the most recent year, the survey captured the current practices of >2000 employers regarding the goals and design of health wellness programs and incentives included in health benefit design. Clearly, the train has left the station. To the extent that there may be 'better practices' and resources for some benefit designs may constitute waste, these programs demand greater evaluation.	Thank you. We have added information related to the Kaiser Family Foundation and Health Research and Educational Trust Employer Health Benefits 2012 Annual Survey in the discussion section.
	Second, the issue of distance as a moderator of the effect of fitness center incentives and use should be expanded more and tailored more for the VA. Specifically, give consideration to the challenges of VA facility-based health promotion programs in the context of large VISN areas. Consider the role of "local" programs that are provided closer to a Veteran's home, or at another Veteran service organization that is closer to them. These still need evaluation but could frame new research questions for VA investigators.	Thank you. We expanded on the issue of distance as relates to VA in the discussion section.
	Third, the discussion of alternative study designs is very good but also general. Consider giving an example of a randomized encouragement trial that blends to generalizability of a pragmatic, whole-population evaluation with the internal validity of randomization. See my comment on the draft. Last, I would recommend a slightly deeper discussion of the need for evaluating both the fitness resource as well as the nature of how fitness center use is encouraged. Behavioral econ studies have shown to some extent that you get what you pay for. In other words, if the incentive is for participation, there is greater participation but not necessarily improved health behavior or outcomes. The nature and direction of the incentive is a critical point of study in the future evaluation of these benefits.	Thank you. We elaborated on the role of incentives and encouragement in the discussion section.

Reviewer	Comment	Response
1	There is a missed opportunity here to underscore the enormity of the issue. The horse is out of the barn and we know very little about the health or economic impacts of these forms of incentives, which could divert limited resources from other areas of employee compensation (e.g. salary, other health benefits, lower premiums). Please see the annual Kaiser Family Foundation Employer Survey. The most recent findings are summarized on the kff website and could help to frame the magnitude of efforts to provide such incentives in the commercial sector.	Thank you. See response to related comments above.
	Cash rewards are currently the most common form of incentive used in the large employer sector to encourage wellness program use. It might be listed here separately from "other economic incentives" (under "Intervention") for this purpose. - add blood lipid control and improved work productivity (reduced absenteeism and presenteeism) to possible intermediate outcomes? - add Non-medical cost reductions to Final Outcomes (again economic impact of work productivity, absence, disability, death, and replacement)?	Thank you. We understand these comments are regarding the framework presented. Figure 1 represents an analytic rather than conceptual framework. As such, the analytic framework is not intended to be a comprehensive representation of all outcomes.
1	There is another opportunity here to relate this to the VA. Because many Veterans travel great distances to access VA facilities, a model that provides or encourages access to peripheral fitness facilities or programs (commercial or through CBOCs or other veteran-accessible organizations such as a VFW) could, in fact, have advantages. This may raise the relevance of encouraging greater research in this area as it may help specifically to serve unique needs of veteran patients.	Thank you. We added details on travel distance for Veterans to the discussion section.
	Might discuss briefly CRET designs. Specifically, pragmatic trials that randomize at the employer level to encouragement versus no encouragement of eligible employees to participate in a physical fitness benefit program. Treatment effects are estimated using an instrumental variables approach that uses random assignment as the instrument. This allows simultaneous assessment of both the encouragement step (interventions may include cash rewards, premium discounts, etc) and use of the fitness facility itself.	Thank you. We added information on the use of incentives as a strategy to increase compliance with the fitness center benefit to the Discussion section.
2	Given that only one cohort of patients was found I agree it is very hard to make any generalizable statements regarding KQ1.	Thank you.
	In consideration of this proposed benefit the key piece of information is how likely people who are not likely to be regularly physically active without the benefit will convert to being physically active with the benefit. If people are already going to fitness clubs, addition of the benefit will not be beneficial. Similar the large number of people with no interest in attending fitness clubs lowers the of health improvement to a population who is offered the benefit change. I understand this is out of scope of this review but does highlight the relevant questions for population health improvement.	Thank you. We agree these are important points to consider, which are further elaborated and addressed in the Discussion section.

Reviewer	Comment	Response
3	I believe it would be helpful to look at Health Service Research Centers associated with health plans and review HEDIS measures of plans that offer gym membership for member utilization and satisfaction, and to see if a retrospective study could be possible using a common methodology across plans for behavioral and health outcomes. Niko Pronk of Health Partners would be a good place to start.	Thank you. This is an excellent idea for future study and one of the study designs addressed in the Recommendations for Future Research.
4	On p. 6, in the Conclusion section, the end of the second sentence indicates the evidence remains "weak". I would recommend changes this statement somewhat to read "…remains insufficient and weak, mostly due to study design limitations and small number of studies that meet criteria for inclusion."	Thank you. These changes were incorporated.
	On p. 8, second paragraph, line 9: I would recommend to insert "full or partial" between the words "providing" and "membership"	

Optional Dissemination and Implementation Questions

Question 5: Are there any clinical performance measures, programs, quality improvement measures, patient care services, or conferences that will be directly affected by this report? If so, please provide detail.

Reviewer	Comment	Response
1	I believe VA National Center for Health Promotion at Durham VA is exploring linkages to outside facilities as a potential means to expand the reach or impact of the MOVE program. Perhaps this is what instigated this particular review in the first place. The review team should be aware of this, but it is worth mentioning.	Thank you.
2	No comment from reviewer 2.	Thank you.
3	No comment from reviewer 3.	Thank you.
4	Unsure as I am not too familiar with the VA programs	Thank you.

Question 6: Please provide any recommendations on how this report can be revised to more directly address or assist implementation needs.

Reviewer	Comment	Response
1	Please see my comments under #4 above, as I believe these also have relevance to implementation needs. However, it is clear that the most direct interpretation of the review is that we currently know very little about the costs and effectiveness of health benefit designs that attempt to improve health through external facility use. The immediate need for implementation seems to be the design of natural experiments that help address this knowledge gap, both within and outside the VA. The review should clearly be framed for the VA research community (and I think it is already) and also designed to engage those investigators with program designers at local VAs or at the National Center.	Thank you. We agree, and the reviewer mentions some next likely steps.
2	No comment from reviewer 2.	Thank you.
3	To encourage future research among those with shared interests by speaking at meetings such as AHIP, YMCA-USA, and health plan health service researchers with health promotion interests.	Thank you. The ESP Coordinating Center dissemination plan includes some or all of the following as applicable: cyberseminar, email distribution, briefing to VA leaders, and manuscript publication.

Effects of Health Plan-Sponsored Fitness Center Benefits

Reviewer	Comment	Response
4	From the systematic review perspective, I don't think there is anything missing. To make the report more directly practical, it may be a good idea to add a series of interviews with health plans that have implemented this type of program to find out what additional analyses they may be using to justify the investment internally. Based on such findings, both a justification for doing this or not may be made as well as a more robust set of information to consider the actual program design elements that may make it a good value for the money.	Thank you. Interviews with health plans may be a direction for future research, but primary data collection is beyond the scope of this review.
Question 7: Please provide us with contact details of any additional individuals/stakeholders who should be made aware of this report.		
1	This should be made accessible to the purchasers (employers, Medicare, and state Medicaid administrators) who are either designing health benefits with public monies or are being asked to purchase such benefits from health plans. The purchasers are looking for answers but are also creating a market demand for these programs with little to know information about whether they work, or how to improve them to work best. This creates waste and could be directing limited resources away from other programs that have greater value for the dollar. Commercial health plans may not be concerned because they are profiting already; why support an evaluation that could show something profitable isn't working? Because of the limited scope and limited information to guide policy changes within the review, this review may be difficult to publish in a scientific journal. However, I would encourage the team try to do this and that distribution to CMMI and to the National Business Group on Health be considered strongly.	Thank you. The ESP Coordinating Center dissemination plan includes some or all of the following as applicable: cyberseminar, email distribution, briefing to VA leaders, and manuscript publication.
2	No comment from reviewer 2.	Thank you.
3	No comment from reviewer 3.	Thank you.
4	I think this report would be of interest to AHIP (America's Health Insurance Plans) and ACHP (the Alliance of Community Health Plans)	Thank you. The ESP Coordinating Center dissemination plan includes some or all of the following as applicable: cyberseminar, email distribution, briefing to VA leaders, and manuscript publication.

APPENDIX E. GLOSSARY

Abstract screening

The stage in a systematic review during which titles and abstracts of articles identified in the literature search are screened for inclusion or exclusion based on established criteria. Articles that pass the abstract screening stage are promoted to the full-text review stage.

Allocation concealment

The method by which randomization assignment is concealed from participants and investigators before and during the enrollment process. Common processes are central allocation (telephone or web-based, pharmacy or off-site statistician controlled randomization sequence generation and sequentially numbered, opaque, sealed envelopes. Allocation concealment concentrates on preventing selection and confounding biases, safeguards the assignment sequence *before and until* allocation, and can always be successfully implemented

Case-control study

A retrospective, analytical, observational study often based on secondary data in which the proportion of cases with a potential risk factor are compared to the proportion of controls (individuals without the disease or condition) with the same risk factor. The common association measure for a case-control study is the odds ratio. These studies are commonly used for initial, inexpensive evaluation of risk factors and are particularly useful for rare conditions or for risk factors with long induction periods. Unfortunately, due to the potential for many forms of bias in this study type, case control studies provide relatively weak empirical evidence even when properly executed.

Case report

A description of a single case, typically describing the manifestations, clinical course, and prognosis of that case. Due to the wide range of natural biologic variability in these aspects, a single case report provides little empirical evidence to the clinician. A case report does describe how others diagnosed and treated the condition and what the clinical outcome was.

Case series

A descriptive, observational study of a series of cases, typically describing the manifestations, clinical course, and prognosis of a condition. A case series provides weak empirical evidence because of the lack of comparability unless the findings are dramatically different from expectations. Case series are best used as a source of hypotheses for investigation by stronger study designs, leading some to suggest that the case series should be regarded as clinicians talking to researchers. Unfortunately, the case series is the most common study type in the clinical literature.

ClinicalTrials.gov

A registry and results database of federally and privately supported clinical trials conducted in the United States and around the world. ClinicalTrials.gov provides information about a trial's purpose, location, participant characteristics, among other details.

Cochrane Database of Systematic Reviews

A bibliographic database of peer-reviewed systematic reviews and protocols prepared by the Cochrane Review Groups in The Cochrane Collaboration.

Cochran's Q test

A nonparametric statistic to test for differences in intervention effects between studies. Because the test statistic is often underpowered, the threshold for statistically significant differences in intervention effects is often set at p<0.10.

Cohort study

A prospective, analytical, observational study based on data, usually primary, from a followup period of a group in which some have had, have, or will have the exposure of interest, to determine the association between that exposure and an outcome. Cohort studies are susceptible to bias by differential loss to followup, the lack of control over risk assignment, and the potential for zero time bias when the cohort is assembled. Because of their prospective nature, cohort studies are stronger than case-control studies when well executed, but they also are more expensive. Because of their observational nature, cohort studies do not provide empirical evidence that is as strong as that provided by properly executed randomized controlled clinical trials.

Companion article

A publication from a trial that is not the article containing the main results of that trial. It may be a methods paper, a report of subgroup analyses, a report of combined analyses, or other auxiliary topic that adds information to the interpretation of the main publication.

Confidence interval (CI)

The range in which a particular result (such as a laboratory test) is likely to occur for everyone in the population of interest a specified percentage of the time known as the confidence level or confidence coefficient. It is an interval calculated from a study's observations used to estimate the reliability of the estimate of a parameter. The most common confidence level is 95%. For example, a confidence interval with a 95% confidence level is intended to give the assurance that, if the statistical model is correct, then taken over all the data that *might* have been obtained, the true value of the parameter will be found within the given interval 95% of the time.

Consistency

The extent to which effect size and direction vary within and across studies; inconsistency may be due to heterogeneity across PICOTS.

Cumulative Index to Nursing and Allied Health Literature (CINAHL)

A collection of medical databases of nursing and allied health literature.

Data abstraction

The stage of a systematic review that involves a pair of trained researchers extracting reported findings specific to the research questions from the full-text articles that met the established inclusion criteria. These data form the basis of the evidence synthesis.

Directness

Degree to which outcomes that are important to users of the comparative effectiveness review (patients, clinicians, or policymakers) are encompassed by trial data.

Embase

A database containing bibliographic records with citations, abstracts, and indexing derived from biomedical and pharmacological articles in peer-reviewed journals.

Exclusion criteria

The criteria, or standards, set out before a study or review. Exclusion criteria are used to determine whether a person should participate in a research study or whether an individual study should be excluded in a systematic review. Exclusion criteria may include age, previous treatments, and other medical conditions.

External validity

The extent to which clinical research studies apply to broader populations. A research study has external validity if its results can be generalized to the larger population.

Forest plot

A visual display of information from individual studies in a meta-analysis. A forest plot shows the amount of variation between the results of the studies as well as an estimate of the overall result of all the studies together. A horizontal line represents the 95% confidence interval (CI) of the "effect" observed in the studies.

Full-text review

The stage of a systematic review in which a pair of trained researchers evaluates the full-text of study articles for potential inclusion in the review.

GRADE

Grading of Recommendations Assessment, Development and Evaluation (GRADE), a systematic approach to evaluating the overall body of research evidence and rating the quality of medical evidence and the strength of clinical recommendations.

Health-related quality of life (HRQOL)

Aspects of overall quality of life that can be clearly shown to affect health—either physical or mental health.

I^2

A statistic that describes the percentage (range from 0–100%) of total variation across studies due to heterogeneity between study characteristics rather than due to chance. Heterogeneity is categorized as low, moderate or high based on I^2 values of 25, 50 or 75%, respectively. It is considered an indication of consistency or inconsistency across studies in a meta-analysis.

Inclusion criteria

The criteria, or standards, set out before the systematic review. Inclusion criteria are used to determine whether an individual study can be included in a systematic review. Inclusion criteria may include population, study design, gender, age, type of disease being treated, previous treatments, and other medical conditions.

Intent-to-treat analysis

A method of analyzing results of a randomized controlled trial that includes in the analysis all cases that should have received a treatment regimen but for some reason did not. All cases allocated to each arm of the trial are analyzed together as representing that treatment arm, regardless of whether they received or completed the prescribed regimen.

Interquartile range (IQR)

A measure of the spread of or dispersion within a data set. The IQR is the width of an interval that contains the middle 50 percent of the sample, so it is smaller than the range and its value is less affected by outliers.

Meta-analysis

A way of combining data from many different research studies. A meta-analysis is a statistical process that combines the findings from individual studies.

Meta-regression analyses

An extension of meta-analysis to subgroups that allows the effect of continuous, as well as categorical, characteristics to be investigated if sufficient studies examining the same characteristics may be compared. In principle, it allows the effect of multiple factors to be investigated simultaneously. In meta-regression, the outcome variable is the effect estimate (e.g., a mean difference, etc.). The explanatory variables are characteristics of studies that might influence the size of the intervention effect.

Mixed effects

Statistical models that include both fixed (nonrandom) and random effects.

Nonrandomized study

Any quantitative study estimating the effectiveness of an intervention (harm or benefit) that does not use randomization to allocate units to comparison groups (including studies where "allocation" occurs in the course of usual treatment decisions or peoples' choices; i.e., studies usually called "observational"). There are many possible types of nonrandomized intervention studies, including cohort studies, case-control studies, controlled before-and-after studies, interrupted-time-series studies, and controlled trials that do not use appropriate randomization strategies (sometimes called quasi-randomized studies).

Observational study

A study in which the investigators do not seek to intervene but simply observe the course of events. Changes or differences in one characteristic (e.g., whether or not people received the intervention of interest) are studied in relation to changes or differences in other characteristics (e.g., whether or not they died), without action by the investigator. Observational studies provide weaker empirical evidence than do experimental studies because of the potential for large confounding biases to be present when there is an unknown association between a factor and an outcome.

Odds ratio

A ratio of the odds of having the outcome of interest in a group with a particular exposure, symptom, or characteristic of interest, to the odds of outcome in a group that does not have the exposure/symptom/characteristic. An odds ratio of 1 indicates that the outcome is equally likely to occur in both groups. An odds ratio of 4 indicates that the outcome is 4 times more likely to be present in the group that has the symptom or characteristic of interest, compared with the group that does not have this symptom. When outcomes are infrequent, the odds ratio is a good approximation of the risk ratio.

PICOTS

Population, intervention, comparator, outcome, timing, setting.

Precision

The degree of certainty for estimate of effect with respect to a specific outcome.

Preferred Reporting Items of Systematic Reviews and Meta-Analyses (PRISMA)

An evidence-based minimum set of items for reporting in systematic reviews and meta-analyses.

Probability

The likelihood (or chance) that an event will occur. In a clinical research study, it is the number of times a condition or event occurs in a study group divided by the number of people being studied.

Prospective observational study

A clinical research study in which people who presently have a certain condition or receive a particular treatment are followed over time and compared with another group of people who are not affected by the condition.

PsycINFO

An abstracting and indexing database of peer-reviewed literature in the behavioral sciences and mental health.

Publication bias

The tendency of researchers to publish experimental findings that have a positive result, while not publishing the findings when the results are negative or inconclusive. The effect of publication bias is that published studies may be misleading. When information that differs from that of the published study is not known, people are able to draw conclusions using only information from the published studies.

PubMed

A database of citations for biomedical literature from MEDLINE, life science journals, and online books in the fields of medicine, nursing, dentistry, veterinary medicine, the health care system, and preclinical sciences.

Quasi-experimental study

A type of study that manipulates a variable between two or more groups, but participants are not randomly assigned to groups. Quasi-experimental study designs, such as nonrandomized pre-post studies, are frequently used when it is not logistically feasible or ethical to conduct a randomized controlled trial.

Randomized controlled trial

A prospective, analytical, experimental study using primary data generated in the clinical environment. Individuals similar at the beginning of the trial are randomly allocated to two or more treatment groups and the outcomes the groups are compared after sufficient followup time. Properly executed, the RCT is the strongest evidence of the clinical efficacy of preventive and therapeutic procedures in the clinical setting.

Relative risk (RR)

A comparison of the risk of a particular event for different groups of people. Relative risk is usually used to estimate exposure to something that could affect health. In a clinical research study, the experimental group is exposed to a particular drug or treatment. The control group is not. The number of events in each group is compared to determine relative risk.

Reporting bias

A bias caused by only a subset of all the relevant data being available. The publication of research can depend on the nature and direction of the study results. Studies in which an intervention is not found to be effective are sometimes not published. Because of this, systematic reviews that fail to include unpublished studies may overestimate the true effect of an intervention. In addition, a published report might present a biased set of results (e.g., only outcomes or subgroups where a statistically significant difference was found).

Risk

A way of expressing the chance that something will happen. It is a measure of the association between exposure to something and what happens (the outcome). Risk is the same as probability, but it usually is used to describe the probability of an adverse event. It is the rate of events (such as breast cancer) in the total population of people who could have the event (such as women of a certain age).

Standard error

The standard deviation of the sampling distribution of a statistic. Measurements taken from a sample of the population will vary from sample to sample. The standard error is a measure of the variation in the sample statistic over all possible samples of the same size. The standard error decreases as the sample size increases.

Standardized mean difference (SMD)

The difference between two estimated means divided by an estimate of the standard deviation. It is used to combine results from studies using different ways of measuring the same concept, e.g. mental health. By expressing the effects as a standardized value, the results can be combined since they have no units.

Statistical significance

A mathematical technique to measure whether the results of a study are likely to be true. Statistical significance is calculated as the probability that an effect observed in a research study is occurring because of chance. Statistical significance is usually expressed as a P-value. The smaller the P-value, the less likely it is that the results are due to chance (and more likely that the results are true). Researchers generally believe the results are probably true if the statistical significance is a P-value less than 0.05 ($p<.05$).

Strength of evidence (SOE)

A measure of how confident reviewers are about decisions that may be made based on a body of evidence. SOE is evaluated using one of four grades: (1) *High* confidence that the evidence reflects the true effect; further research is very unlikely to change reviewer confidence in the estimate of effect; (2) *moderate* confidence that the evidence reflects the true effect; further research may change the confidence in the estimate of effect and may change the estimate; (3) *low* confidence that the evidence reflects the true effect; further research is likely to change the confidence in the estimate of effect and is likely to change the estimate; and (4) *insufficient*; the evidence either is unavailable or does not permit a conclusion.

Systematic review

A summary of the clinical literature. A systematic review is a critical assessment and evaluation of all research studies that address a particular clinical issue. The researchers use an organized method of locating, assembling, and evaluating a body of literature on a particular topic using a set of specific criteria. A systematic review typically includes a description of the findings of the collection of research studies. The systematic review may also include a quantitative pooling of data, called a meta-analysis.

Time-series study

A quasi-experimental research design in which periodic measurements are made on a defined group of individuals both before and after implementation of an intervention. Time series studies are often conducted for the purpose of determining the intervention or treatment effect.

www.ingramcontent.com/pod-product-compliance
Lightning Source LLC
Chambersburg PA
CBHW081624170526
45166CB00009B/3097